THE LEAKY GUT MEAL PLAN

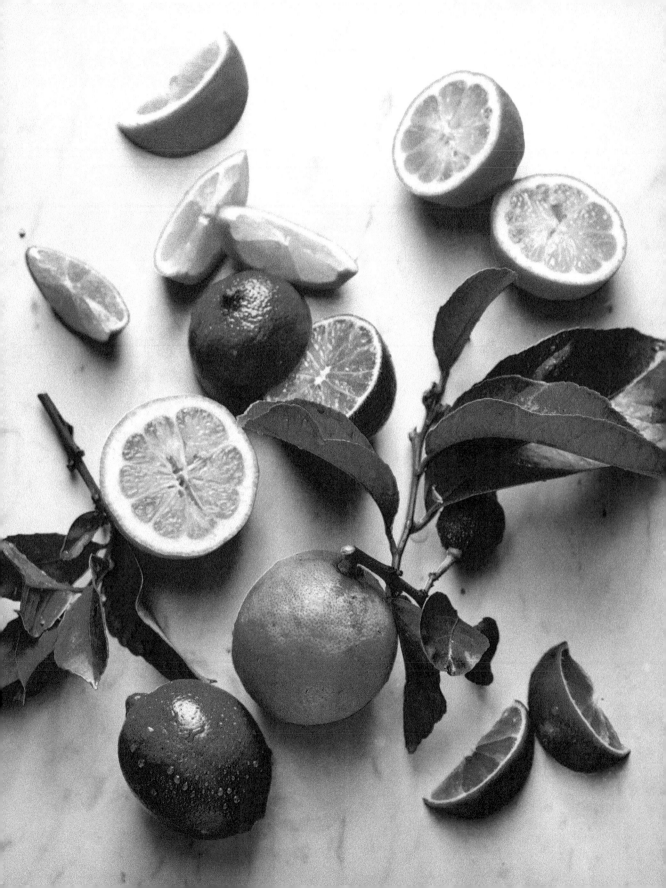

THE LEAKY GUT
MEAL PLAN

4 WEEKS to Detox and Improve Digestive Health

SARAH KAY HOFFMAN

ROCKRIDGE
PRESS

Interior and Cover Designer: Diana Haas
Photo Art Director: Hillary Frileck
Editor: Barbara J. Isenberg
Production Manager: Holly Haydash
Photography © 2019 Andrew Purcell, Food styling by Carrie Purcell, Photography © Nadine Greeff p. viii
Author photo courtesy of © 2019 Makayla Rae Photography

ISBN: Print 978-1-64152-884-9 | eBook 978-1-64152-885-6
R0

To the Gutsy community:

When you heal your gut, you heal your life.

Never give up hope that your best days are yet to come.

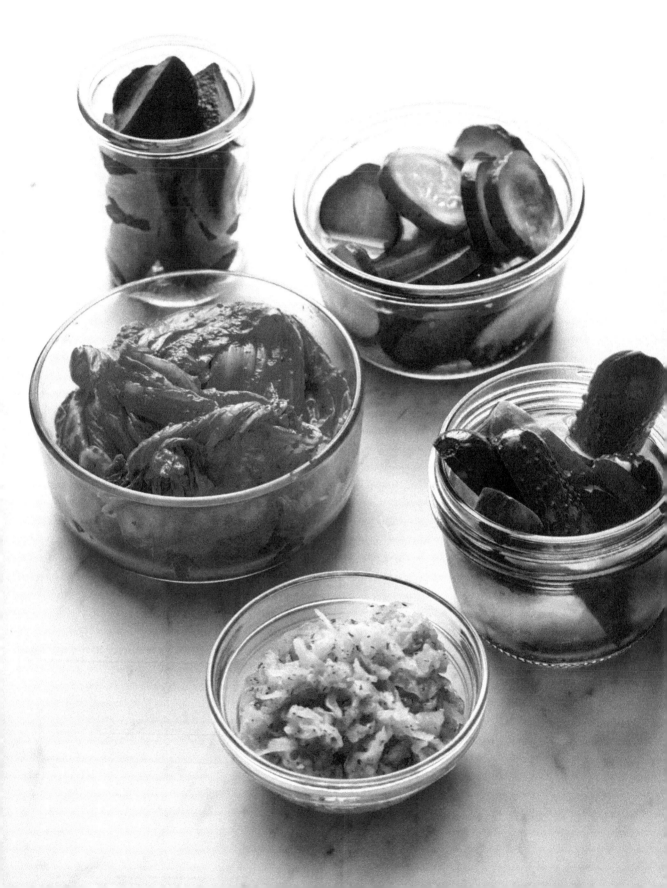

CONTENTS

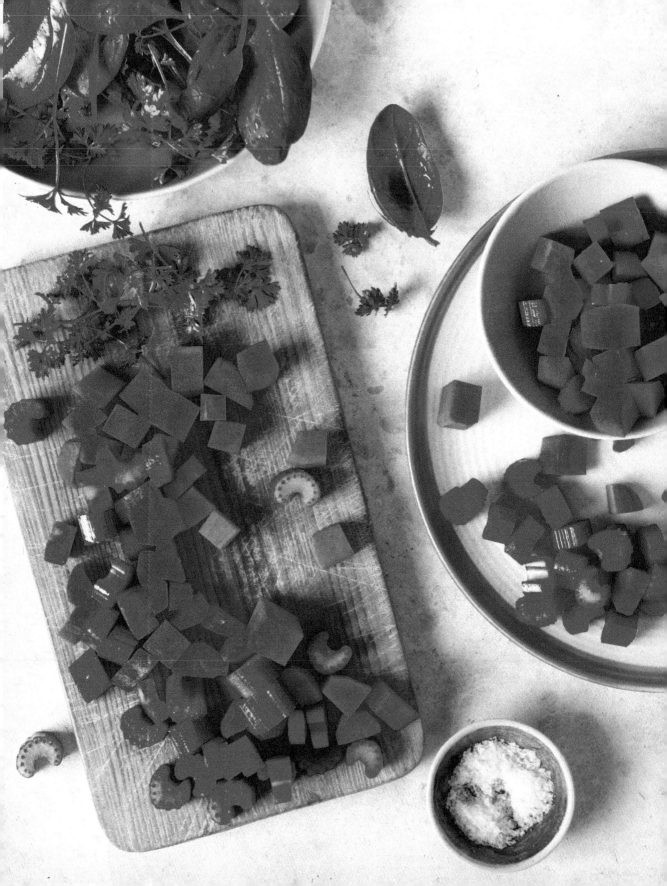

INTRODUCTION

If you are holding this book, it's likely you (or someone you love) are struggling with a variety of digestive and other issues and can't seem to make any progress in healing. I'm here to tell you from personal experience that there is hope!

My name is Sarah Kay Hoffman, but to those in the gut-healing community, I am *A Gutsy Girl*. That's the name of the online community I founded in 2012 to help women worldwide connect and support one another in our healing journeys. I believe in the power that gut healing has on overall health and on our entire lives, and I am an avid and passionate gut health researcher and journalist.

At one point or another in my life, I was diagnosed with ulcerative colitis, irritable bowel syndrome, a low-functioning thyroid, "adrenal fatigue," and more. In 2009, I did a food intolerance test, and the results showed that I was intolerant to 22 different foods, including egg white, dairy milk, shrimp, lentils, and celery. There wasn't any pattern, so I just worked very hard to avoid all of them.

I proceeded to go through blood testing, stool sample testing, colonoscopies, and endoscopies. I tried medications, herbal remedies, supplements, and dietary changes. I went to countless doctors and followed different protocols.

Years later, I discovered that I had leaky gut syndrome. So I wasn't necessarily intolerant to all of those foods; rather, my gut had become "leaky," which caused my body to react to those foods and so many more. At last, something that made sense!

In this book, I present my 4-week meal plan to help you get on the right track for gut health, which can improve your overall health. There is no better time to heal your gut and your life than today. My hope is that you will be on your forever path to ultimate gut health and healing during these next few weeks.

EGGS AND GREENS BUDDHA
BOWL, PAGE 71

PART ONE

To Better Gut Health

Before we turn to a recipe plan to help you heal your gut issues, let's first take a few minutes to explore how the gut works. Then we'll look at what leaky gut syndrome is, how it impacts overall health, and how changes in both diet and lifestyle can reverse the effects of leaky gut syndrome. The more you understand, the more likely you are to take action, and action is the *only* way you can truly start healing.

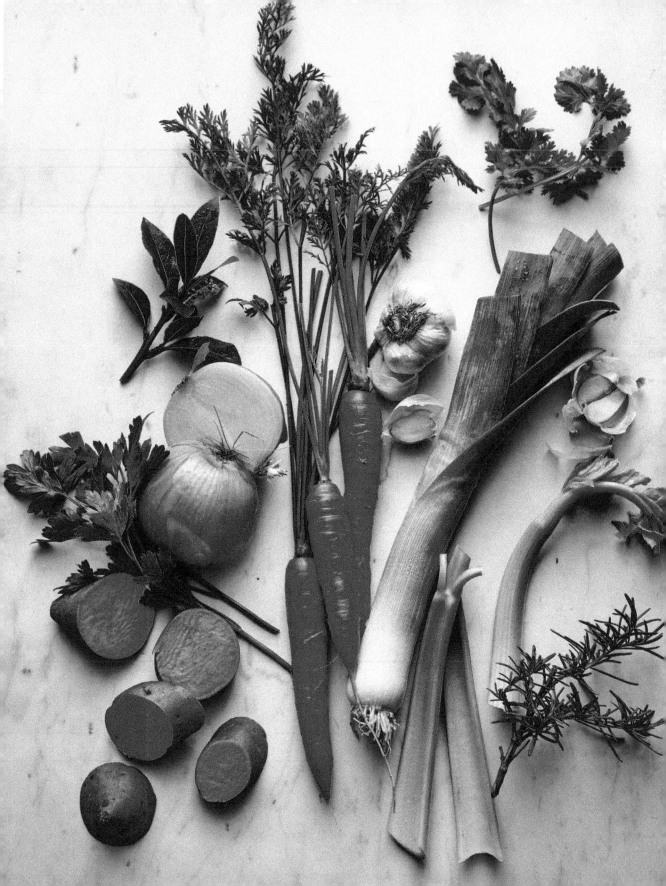

CHAPTER ONE

Understanding Your Gut

More than two thousand years ago, the Greek physician Hippocrates stated, "All disease begins in the gut." As modern medical research increasingly demonstrates that he was right, more and more people have become interested in the idea that their gut health is closely linked to their overall health.

In your car, your tire might have a slow leak that you don't even notice, but you can be sure that it will eventually lead to a flat tire. In the same way, the absence of illness in your body doesn't automatically mean that you are healthy. But like a trickle effect, when one medical issue presents itself, so might another, then another.

WHAT IS LEAKY GUT SYNDROME?

You might have heard the term *leaky gut syndrome*, but what exactly is it? Simply put, leaky gut syndrome (also known as intestinal permeability) is a condition in which the cells that make up the lining of the small intestine become so inflamed that the lining becomes more permeable, or porous, than it's meant to be. When this happens, foreign substances can enter the bloodstream, causing the body's immune system to shift into reaction mode by creating antibodies against its own tissues.

How a Healthy Gut Works

To help us better understand leaky gut syndrome, let's first look at the process of digestion in its most basic form.

The entire digestive system contains 10 organs, with more than 20 specialized cell types, making it one of the most diverse and complicated systems in the entire body. The gastrointestinal (GI) tract occupies 300 to 400 square feet in your body. It runs from the mouth to the anus through a series of hollow organs: the esophagus, stomach, small intestine, and large intestine.

The GI tract not only breaks down food, absorbs nutrients and water, and removes waste products but also acts as a barrier between your gut and bloodstream to prevent harmful substances from entering your body.

The digestive system breaks down nutrients into small enough parts for the body to absorb and use for energy, growth, and cell repair. The intestines have small gaps that allow nutrients and water to pass into your bloodstream. In a healthy gut, these gaps are very small in order to prevent potentially harmful substances like bacteria, toxins, and undigested food particles from entering the bloodstream.

Healthy guts move food through the GI tract through a process called peristalsis, which is a wavelike movement that helps push food along. In addition to peristalsis, chewing, saliva, digestive juices, stomach acid, bile, and enzymes also help with digestion. Furthermore, inside the GI tract, there are a variety of bacteria that can be both helpful and harmful to the digestive process. The bacteria are also known as gut flora, or an individual's microbiome.

Food usually stays in the stomach for about three hours, then moves to the small intestine. In the small intestine, most of the nutrients from food become absorbed, and special cells help these absorbed nutrients cross the intestinal lining into your bloodstream. They are then delivered to the rest of the body.

Digestion is completed when leftover fiber, water, and dead cells head to the large intestine (also known as the colon). The body drains out most of the remaining fluid through the intestinal wall. The final product left is stool, which the colon squeezes through to the rectum. Nerves expand in the rectum, ultimately excreting the final waste through the anus.

This entire process, from eating to excreting, takes 30 to 40 hours to complete.

Signs of a Healthy Gut

How do you know if your gut is working as it should? Here are some signs:

- You are able to tolerate foods that are considered harder to digest, like raw fruits and vegetables.

- You are not often sick, suggesting that your immune system is functioning optimally.

- You have few (if any) food sensitivities or intolerances.

- Your bowel movements happen regularly and are solid.

- You have no bloating or constipation.

- Your skin is clear.

You could spend your entire life wondering whether or not your gut is healthy—whether or not you are healthy. But the only way of knowing for sure is through testing, not guessing. Tests for zonulin, IgG food intolerance, and vitamin and mineral deficiencies can help determine whether your gut is leaky, as can testing with lactulose.

When a Gut Is Leaky

When there is an increase in the permeability of the intestinal mucosa, bacteria, toxic digestive metabolites, bacterial toxins, and small molecules can "leak" into the bloodstream. In simpler terms, what is supposed to be a tight barrier, controlling what gets through to the bloodstream, becomes looser or develops large cracks or holes, making it easier for harmful substances to penetrate the tissue beneath it.

Signs of a Leaky Gut

Leaky gut can present itself in many different ways, and it varies from person to person. Some symptoms may not even be related to the location they are associated with. For example, if you have acne, the root cause may be your gut and not your skin!

Here are some signs that your gut might be leaky:

- Digestive symptoms, including gas, bloating, constipation, or diarrhea

- Seasonal allergies or asthma

- Hormonal imbalances

- Autoimmune disease, such as lupus or multiple sclerosis

- Chronic fatigue syndrome or fibromyalgia

- Mood and cognitive issues, such as ADD, ADHD, and "brain fog"

- Skin issues, such as acne and rosacea

- Candida overgrowth

- Food allergies and intolerances

- Inflammatory bowel disease (IBD)—ulcerative colitis and Crohn's disease

- Celiac disease

- Irritable bowel syndrome (IBS)

- Headaches

- Gastric ulcers

- Acute inflammation, such as sepsis, the body's extreme response to infection

- Chronic inflammation, such as arthritis

- Obesity-associated metabolic diseases, such as type 2 diabetes

According to current medical thinking, leaky gut does not cause these conditions. Rather, those with leaky gut are more likely to have any number of other problems, including the ones described above, occurring simultaneously. Therefore, it is believed that leaky gut syndrome is in fact a symptom of something larger.

The research world is booming today with studies suggesting that both inflammation and modifications in intestinal bacteria may play a role in the development of several common chronic diseases. What is certain is that by eating a nutritious, unprocessed diet, inflammation can be reduced, which, in turn, can help rebuild the gut lining and bring balance to the gut flora.

Causes of Leaky Gut

You're probably wondering what caused your leaky gut. Again, everyone is different, but here are some of the most commonly discussed causes:

ALCOHOL. Although you can find studies showing that low levels of alcohol are good for the brain, most studies now demonstrate that there's no amount of alcohol consumption that's good for overall health. Furthermore, when it comes to the gut, research shows that alcohol promotes bacterial overgrowth, which in turn leads to an increase in the release of endotoxins. Endotoxins activate proteins and immune system cells that promote inflammation.

CERTAIN PAINKILLERS AND NONSTEROIDAL ANTI-INFLAMMATORY DRUGS (NSAIDS). The job of an NSAID is to relieve inflammation, which it does by blocking an enzyme called cyclooxygenase. However, when this enzyme is blocked, it's not available to perform important functions like protecting the stomach from its own acid and strengthening the activity of the immune system. Among people who chronically use NSAIDs, research estimates that 65 percent will develop intestinal inflammation and up to 30 percent will develop ulcers. Eventually, these conditions could lead to autoimmune disease.

ANTIBIOTICS. There's no question that antibiotics are absolutely critical for treating certain infections and can even be lifesaving. However, antibiotics work by wiping out all bacteria—whether good or bad—so beneficial and protective gut bacteria are compromised. Furthermore, overuse of antibiotics may leave the strong and drug-resistant bacteria behind to colonize the digestive system and exacerbate leaky gut syndrome.

PREEXISTING CONDITIONS. Researchers haven't concluded whether preexisting conditions like inflammatory bowel disease, gut infections, diabetes, and complicated surgeries cause the gut to be leaky or whether a leaky gut leads to these conditions. What is certain, though, is that preexisting conditions are usually found in conjunction with leaky gut.

PROCESSED FOODS. There is emerging evidence that the standard American diet (SAD), which is low in fiber and high in sugar and saturated fats, may trigger a leaky gut scenario. Additionally, many processed foods are inflammatory and high in allergens such as gluten and dairy, not to mention an abundance of sugar, refined oils, and artificial preservatives.

CHRONIC STRESS. Chronic stress is a major player in leaky gut, weakening the immune system and contributing to anxiety and depression. Some stress is completely natural and normal; ongoing stress is damaging.

TOXINS. The body encounters toxins every day, in many different forms. Toxins can be present in our food (such as many of the foods we will be eliminating in the 4-week leaky gut meal plan), air, water, home (such as mold), and even clothing. We can never completely avoid toxins, but when too many of them build up and cannot be eliminated appropriately, they cause damage to the body, including to the gut.

GRAINS AND GLUTEN. Gluten is believed to trigger leaky gut syndrome in individuals genetically predisposed to celiac disease. But even if you do not have celiac disease, eating grains can cause damage to your gut. Grains contain lectins and phytates, so-called antinutrients that bind to the intestines and make nutrients inactive in the body. Furthermore, traditionally processed grains and GMOs (genetically modified organisms) often contain heavy pesticides, high levels of mycotoxins (toxic substances produced by a fungus), and mold, all of which wreak havoc on the gut.

"TOO CLEAN" OF AN ENVIRONMENT. Wait a minute, too clean? Yes, it's true, the fear of getting sick from germs may actually be causing an increased prevalence of leaky gut syndrome. Overuse of antibacterial cleaning products and hand sanitizers wipes out all the beneficial good bacteria we need to fight off unwanted bacteria and illness.

GENETIC PREDISPOSITION. Some people may be predisposed to leaky gut because they are sensitive to environmental factors that can trigger the body into initiating an autoimmune response.

The Connection to Autoimmune Conditions

When toxic substances and undigested fats and proteins leak from the GI tract into the bloodstream, they attach themselves to various tissues throughout the body. The body then produces antibodies, triggering an allergic response that creates inflammation and damages tissues and organs.

If this condition lasts only a short period of time, it is not likely to cause health problems. But when the immune system is constantly in overdrive, with time it becomes highly reactive, responding to stimuli that it would have previously ignored, which keeps the intestinal gates open and inflammation building.

As inflammation builds, it can lead to the development of many autoimmune conditions. Wherever the inflammation is triggered, that's where the autoimmunity occurs: if it's the joints, rheumatoid arthritis; if it's the lungs, asthma; if it's the gut lining, ulcerative colitis or Crohn's disease.

Some of the major autoimmune conditions that have been associated with leaky gut syndrome include type 1 diabetes, lupus, inflammatory bowel disease (IBD: ulcerative colitis and Crohn's disease), celiac disease, autoimmune hepatitis, multiple sclerosis, psoriatic arthritis, Hashimoto's thyroiditis, Sjögren's syndrome, fibromyalgia, and psoriasis.

Because of the strong connection between leaky gut syndrome and autoimmune conditions, if you have been diagnosed with an autoimmune condition, you would likely need to take the 4-week leaky gut syndrome meal plan a step further. This is discussed in chapter 2 (page 46).

HOW LEAKY GUT AFFECTS THE BODY

Having a leaky gut means that harmful substances like bacteria, toxins, and undigested food particles can enter the bloodstream, so the gut is far from the only system affected. Indeed, leaky gut affects every part of the body.

Symptoms like bloating, diarrhea, menstrual irregularities, and frequent colds are common. Those symptoms also often lead to other diagnoses, such as IBS, IBD, thyroid dysfunction, acne, and more.

In this section, we will go into more detail about the symptoms of leaky gut and how leaky gut affects the body and overall health.

Brain

Clear correlations have been discovered between gut dysfunction and autism, dyspraxia, ADD, ADHD, dyslexia, depression, and schizophrenia. Could this also align with the fact that 95 percent of serotonin, the "happy neurotransmitter," is made and stored in your gut?

On a more relatable level, certain situations make us feel nauseated or give us "butterflies" in our stomach. Ever had that "gut feeling"? All of this exemplifies the gut-brain connection.

Since millions of nerves and neurons run between your gut and brain, it's no surprise that keeping a diet filled with foods that boost gut health (omega-3 fatty acids, fermented foods, probiotics, and more) can have direct positive effects on the brain. The vagus nerve is one of the largest nerves that send signals along the gut-brain axis. It works in conjunction with enteroendocrine cells in the small intestine to regulate both stress and gastrointestinal issues.

Digestive System

The most common place people expect leaky gut symptoms to show up is the digestive system. Indeed, it is quite uncommon to have leaky gut syndrome and not present any digestive problems.

Digestive symptoms are typically the main reason people suspect they have leaky gut syndrome. The most common GI symptoms are bloating, constipation, and diarrhea. From time to time we all experience a stomachache or other digestive problem, and women tend to feel bloated at certain times during the menstrual cycle. But when these symptoms happen frequently (usually daily), it could be a sign of leaky gut.

Hormones

If you are a woman, perhaps you have experienced unexplained weight loss or weight gain, excessive sweating, difficulty falling or staying asleep, changes in sensitivity to cold and heat, dry skin or skin rashes, increased or decreased blood pressure, heart rate changes, weak bones, irritability or anxiety, unexplained and long-term fatigue, increased thirst, infertility, puffy face, or deepening of the voice.

While these symptoms could be indicative of other issues, they often point to hormonal issues. Finding and addressing the root cause of a hormonal imbalance is the most important step in treating it. And when we do the detective work, it almost always comes back to the gut.

When hormonal symptoms are present, patients might be diagnosed with polycystic ovary syndrome (PCOS), over- or underactive thyroid, endometriosis, or even breast, cervical, or ovarian cancer.

Immune System

The key to overall health is contained within our immune system because it helps protect us from bacteria and other invaders. The immune system also impacts every other system in the body.

An impaired immune system could be the result of an autoimmune condition with more serious symptoms, but it can also result in common, everyday symptoms and illnesses such as muscle pain, frequent colds, and headaches.

Coming down with the common cold is bound to happen to all of us, but those with a weakened immune system have more than the average number of immune system-related issues. You simply cannot be healthy without having a strong gut. If the gut lining is compromised, more illness is almost certainly imminent.

Infections

It is unclear whether leaky gut syndrome makes one more susceptible to other infections of the gut, or having these infections is in fact the cause of leaky gut, but the two do seem to be connected.

The most common causes of GI infection are candida overgrowth, small intestinal bacterial overgrowth (SIBO), and intestinal parasites. There are also other less common causes, such as Epstein-Barr virus (EBV) and Lyme disease.

GI infections come with symptoms like constipation, diarrhea, food intolerances, skin issues, bloating, nutritional deficiencies, joint pain, fatigue, brain fog, sugar cravings, and more. When any of these infections are not addressed, over time they tend to lead to a leaky gut, or leaky gut can lead to them.

Metabolism

If you are suffering from chronic health problems like insulin resistance and metabolic dysfunction, along with abdominal obesity and type 2 diabetes, leaky gut syndrome might be a huge part of the equation.

Having healthy gut bacteria is crucial to maintaining a normal weight and functional metabolism. With leaky gut syndrome, though, inflammation is out of control, and this inflammation is associated with metabolic issues like weight gain and diabetes.

Three separate but related mechanisms have been identified: gut dysbiosis, an unhealthy dietary pattern, and specific nutrient deficiencies. These three risk factors likely interact to cause intestinal permeability and promote the development of metabolic syndrome and obesity.

There isn't a conclusive answer as to whether changes in gut health are the cause or consequence of metabolic dysfunction, but there is certainly a correlation between the two.

Nutrients

If you've recently had a complete blood panel done and were found to be deficient in certain nutrients—typically vitamin A, vitamin B12, vitamin D, magnesium, zinc, iron, and calcium—it maybe be a sign of leaky gut. Nutritional deficiencies may occur even if you consume a relatively nutritious diet because the small intestine is unable to absorb the vitamins and minerals for use in the body.

Without absorbing these (and other) critical nutrients, you're likely to experience overall inflammation and chronic fatigue as well as symptoms specific to the nutrient deficiency—for example, constipation due to magnesium deficiency, brittle bones due to calcium deficiency, and skin issues due to vitamin A deficiency.

Skin

Leaky gut often triggers inflammatory dermatological issues. Most people with leaky gut don't get just an occasional breakout but mild to severe acne. Other skin issues that often present with leaky gut include atopic dermatitis, perioral dermatitis, eczema, and psoriasis.

EATING YOUR WAY TO A HEALTHY GUT

It's been said that we are what we eat. But we are not only what we eat; we are also what we absorb and digest. If the gut is leaky, we can't absorb and digest properly; but if we're not focusing on the right foods and diet in the first place, the gut will become leaky.

Diet is important prior to illness, and it is critical once illness is present because the food we choose to eat (or not eat) will help or hurt the healing process.

One way to help zone in on what foods are or are not working for you is through the use of a food journal. By keeping a record of what foods you're eating, you'll be able to track how those foods make you feel—physically and emotionally—on a daily basis.

Eat Healthy Fats

In decades past, it was thought that fat was something to be avoided in a healthy diet. We now know that this is entirely untrue. In fact, both sugar addiction and the American obesity epidemic began soon after low-fat diets became the standard recommendation.

Eating healthy fats is critical for overall gut health. Healthy fats come from avocados, organic butter and ghee, coconut oil, extra-virgin olive oil, omega-3s (from such foods as salmon, sardines, and walnuts), nuts and seeds, eggs, grass-fed organic beef, organic full-fat dairy, and even dark chocolate (at least 85 percent cacao).

Healthy fats help heal the gut in a variety of ways. For example, extra-virgin olive oil is high in antioxidants, which means it helps protect cells from damage. It also works as an anti-inflammatory, and with leaky gut syndrome, reducing inflammation is key. Grass-fed organic beef contains conjugated linoleic acid, which helps prevent diseases, like diabetes, that often go hand in hand with leaky gut syndrome. Omega-3 fatty acids have been shown to relieve inflammation and reduce symptoms of autoimmune conditions like rheumatoid arthritis, psoriasis, and Crohn's disease.

Drink Stocks and Broths

There's a South American proverb that says, "Good broth will resurrect the dead." Indeed, broth is one of the most important foods for gut healing.

One key to extracting as much intestinal healing benefits from stocks and broths as possible is that they must be animal-based. The gelatin, which is in the thick layer of fat that sits on top of homemade stocks and broths, comes directly from bones. And this gelatin is where the magic is hidden. Gelatin has the ability to calm and soothe, provides an immune system boost, and is nutrient dense.

Vegetable broths absolutely have a place in healing leaky gut, but you'll need a high-quality bone broth in order to get that all-important gelatin for nourishing the intestinal lining and reducing inflammation.

Seek Out "Clean" Meat

Not all meat is created equal. "Clean" is a subjective term, but in this case, we're talking about meat that has not been pumped full of hormones and antibiotics. However, these days most meat is.

If you're eating meat from animals that were fed hormones and antibiotics, you're ingesting them as well. (Remember: You are what you eat.) If you consume antibiotic-laced meat, you will end up with some of the drugs, as well as the resistant bacteria, in your own digestive tract, with potentially harmful results.

Furthermore, antibiotics can disrupt the gut microbiome. The microbiome is key for properly digesting food and processing fats, and alterations or disruptions to it as well as the intestinal lining can cause leaky gut syndrome.

Ferment Your Vegetables

The process of fermenting vegetables has been used for thousands of years in cultures worldwide as a way to preserve food safely. The process of fermentation allows vegetables to sit and steep until their sugars are broken down to promote the growth of probiotics, which are live bacteria and yeasts that help foster a healthy balance of gut bacteria.

Some common fermented vegetable dishes are sauerkraut, pickles, and kimchi (a spicy Korean mix).

In addition to fermented vegetables, other fermented foods also provide these probiotics to support the gut. They include things like yogurt, miso, tempeh, kombucha, and kefir.

Try Cultured Dairy

Cultured dairy is fermented by bacterial cultures that help maintain a healthy gut environment and aid in digestion. It is a low-sugar, high-protein alternative to conventional dairy and is suitable for those who are lactose intolerant.

It's best to eat cultured dairy products as soon as possible after they are produced, before the beneficial bacteria are depleted or become inactive. You can buy cultured dairy products, but you can also make them on your own. It's very simple, and later in the recipe section, you'll learn exactly how to do it (see the recipe for Coconut Yogurt on page 57).

Go Gluten-Free

It is possible that gluten is the number one culprit behind leaky gut. The reason is zonulin, a protein that is released in the intestines and tells the gut lining to "open up." It is believed that in some people, gluten triggers the release of zonulin.

In addition to the zonulin factor, the hybridized wheat we're eating today is not the same as it was in the past. It's estimated that 5 percent of the proteins found in hybridized wheat are new proteins, which have led to increased systemic inflammation and gluten intolerance.

Gluten is in many packaged products, from soups and sauces to cookies, cake, pasta, bread, and more. Beware that if a package says "wheat-free," it's not necessarily gluten-free, because gluten can be found in other grains as well, such as rye and barley. In general, always check ingredient packaging for gluten-free labeling in order to ensure foods, especially oats, were processed in a completely gluten-free facility.

Avoid Sugar

Americans' sugar addiction is making us overweight and lethargic—and destroying our most prized possession, the gut. Excess sugar intake can prevent the small intestine from acting as a barrier, leading to many gastrointestinal disorders, including constipation and poor overall gut function.

If you think artificial sugars like aspartame, sucralose, saccharine, neotame, advantame, and acesulfame potassium are any better, reconsider. In fact, it's been shown that consumption of artificial sweeteners may adversely affect gut microbial activity, which can cause a wide range of health issues, including leaky gut.

While healing leaky gut, it's best to limit the amount of sugar in your daily diet. Some of the sweeteners you can still incorporate in small amounts are raw honey, maple syrup, stevia, coconut sugar, and monk fruit.

Eliminate Genetically Modified Foods

Genetically modified organisms (GMOs) are those that have been modified in a laboratory using genetic engineering or transgenic technology. Some of the most common foods containing GMOs are soy, corn, canola oil, milk, beet sugar, aspartame, zucchini, yellow squash, and papaya.

GMO foods have been shown to potentially cause gastrointestinal damage—including leaky gut—because the immune system does not understand what it's facing (the molecules aren't recognized). This leads to an inflammatory response. The more the intestinal wall is weakened by inflammation, the more "foreign invaders" get through its border.

Whenever possible, look for the "Non-GMO Project Verified" seal on a food product. This official seal means that the product has gone through an extensive verification process.

Avoid Processed and Packaged Foods

Processed foods contribute to inflammation and disrupt food digestion. They are often stripped of valuable vitamins, minerals, and other nutrients and then pumped full of artificial additives your body doesn't need or doesn't know how to process. In addition, some of these additives cause reactions by irritating nerve endings in different parts of the body, in much the same way that certain drugs can cause side effects in sensitive people. This can result in the development of a new food intolerance.

Some of the food additives that can trigger leaky gut or exacerbate symptoms include transglutaminases ("meat glue," found in processed meats), added sugars, and emulsifiers like polysorbate 80 and carboxymethylcellulose.

SUPPLEMENTS FOR GUT HEALTH

Rebuilding the gut lining often requires the use of specific supplements, which is best coordinated along with your health practitioner. When choosing a supplement, be sure you know and trust the source. Many supplements contain additives and fillers, and sometimes the source of the main ingredient is not as high-quality as you think.

Here are some supplements that are believed to help heal the gut:

- **HCl (BETAINE) WITH PEPSIN.** This helps support healthy stomach acidity, gastric function, and protein digestion. Without adequate stomach acid, vitamins and minerals are not absorbed properly, and protein becomes harder to digest. Take only with higher-protein meals.
- **DIGESTIVE ENZYMES.** These support optimal digestion by helping the body absorb nutrients and convert food into energy. They can help with gas, bloating, indigestion, and irregularity.
- **L-GLUTAMINE.** This is an essential amino acid that is anti-inflammatory and necessary for the growth and repair of your intestinal lining. L-glutamine coats the cell walls, acting as a repellent to irritants.
- **DIGESTIVE BITTERS.** These are made of herbs, bark, roots, and fruit and are used to improve digestion and breakdown of fats, reduce gas and bloating, and even help prevent SIBO and yeast overgrowth.
- **ZINC.** This mineral is known for its ability to boost the immune system and help tighten the junctions of the intestinal lining.
- **PROBIOTICS.** These help improve the overall microbiome of the gut by restoring beneficial bacteria that have been depleted.

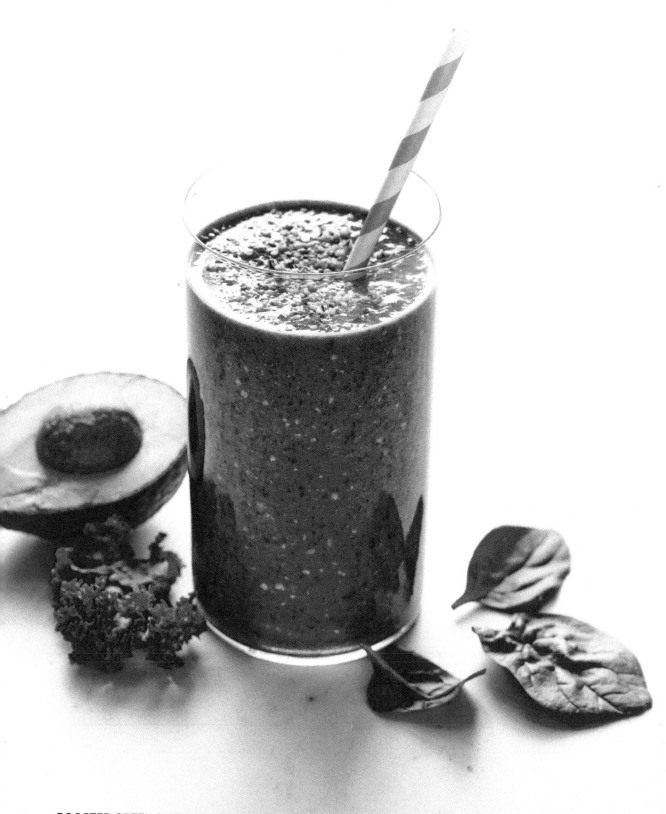

BOOSTED GREEN SMOOTHIE, PAGE 72

CHAPTER TWO

The 4-Week Plan

Now that we've seen how the gut works and looked at some general guidelines for optimal gut health, you're probably wondering, "So what should I eat?"

If you are sick and tired of feeling sick and tired, you're likely ready to make a change with your diet. Doing and eating the same old things will yield the same old results. In order to determine whether a change can help you start feeling better, you'll need to do things and eat in a new way.

But you're ready for it—you've come this far, realizing that nothing changes if nothing changes. These next four weeks will heal your leaky gut in four stages: remove, replace, repair, and rebalance. Each week of the meal plan is focused on one of these steps.

SNAPSHOT OF THE PLAN

The gut is incredibly resilient. In fact, changes can happen within months, weeks, or even days. Yes, days! Knowing this fact should give you all the inspiration and motivation you need to start make long-lasting healing happen.

The purpose of going through a 4-week time line is that it allows the body to rest and reset, then repair and move forward. During this time, our goal is to address dietary and lifestyle areas for improvement, normalize digestion and absorption, begin discovering correlations between dietary and lifestyle decisions, normalize the balance of gut bacteria, and promote overall gastrointestinal healing.

This time line and meal plan will work for anyone who:

- has concerns about leaky gut

- wants to maintain a healthy intestinal lining

- has present or past digestive issues

- needs to repair after a course of antibiotics

- wants to support a healthy immune system

- is ready to beat sugar cravings in order to support a healthy weight

Each weeklong phase of the meal plan has a specific purpose: removing foods, then replacing them, repairing the gut lining, and finally rebalancing it all. By focusing on something different each week, you will start to reset and repair your gut lining and heal your leaky gut.

To start, in week 1, we'll remove all foods that are not beneficial to the digestive system. This phase is similar to a traditional elimination diet in that it will help you understand what is causing your GI and other symptoms. Anything that has the potential to negatively affect the environment of the GI tract will be removed. Some of these include common food allergens (or foods known to cause reactions or sensitivities), food toxins, caffeine, and alcohol.

During week 2, we will begin replacing the digestive secretions that may have been depleted (by diet, antacids or other drugs, disease, or aging) with enzymes, bile salts, and hydrochloric acid that might be lacking in your gut but are essential to proper digestion.

By the time week 3 rolls around, you'll be ready to repair your gut with beneficial bacteria to help regain a healthy microflora balance while supplying it with key nutrients. Probiotic and prebiotic foods will be instrumental for both repairing and beginning to repopulate these beneficial bacteria.

Finally, during week 4, we will focus on rebalancing by paying attention to lifestyle elements (sleep, exercise, stress) while continuing to incorporate all of the critical pieces from the first three weeks. Prebiotic and probiotic foods and supplements are a focal point during this week as well. This is the week when you are likely to begin feeling the positive effects of the program.

While the 4-week meal plan does remove many harmful things from the diet, it can't possibly remove everything that every person may need removed for their own healing journey. This is because at some point, removing too many things can also become problematic for the various systems throughout the body.

This 4-week meal plan includes eggs, nuts, some nightshades (tomatoes and bell peppers, but not potatoes), fruit, FODMAPs (fermentable oligo-, di-, mono-saccharides, and polyols), and a few natural sugars (coconut sugar and honey).

Not all foods are right for everyone, because every food has unique properties that interact in a specific way with the person consuming it. What might be a "yes" food for someone could be a clear "no" for someone else. These next four weeks are sure to start giving you some answers about what works and doesn't work for your body.

Although this is a 4-week meal plan, some people will need (or choose) to stay on this path for far longer. Depending on the current state of your gut, you might need up to six months, or even longer in severe cases, to arrive at a place where you feel healed. The good news is that the recipes contained in this book are so delicious, you're not likely to ever get tired of them!

Take deep breaths, enjoy your food, and embrace the process. It's your time to move forward, make big changes, and have your gut feel better than it ever has before.

WEEK 1: REMOVE

During week 1, the goal is to remove every food (and other factors) that could potentially be harming your gut lining and causing it to be leaky. We do this first and foremost not only to rid your body of all the things that contribute to your pain and misery but also to create space for new, beneficial bacteria. Then you'll be ready to move forward by reintroducing foods slowly and methodically to figure out what you are actually intolerant to and what you can safely still eat. (This, of course, is the best part.)

The major foods we will remove in week 1 are wheat, gluten, grains, corn, non-fermented soy, GMOs, legumes, caffeine, alcohol, processed and packaged foods, refined sugars, refined oils, and dairy. Eggs will be limited.

In addition, we will focus on removing chronic stress; overuse of antibacterial products; and toxic exposure from conventional diets, tap water, pesticides, skincare products, chemicals from plastic, and NSAIDs. You may have read that you should also ditch any antibiotics, but it depends on why they were prescribed, so go with your doctor's recommendation for antibiotics and other medications.

Broths are included in the entire 4-week plan, but they are focused on most during week 1. In fact, many people even choose to do a broth fasting, which consists of anywhere from 24 to 72 hours of sipping solely on broth. We will not do that here, but drinking as much broth as possible throughout the day is an important part of the week 1 meal plan. For this reason, you should plan to have on hand Beef Bone Broth (page 54), Chicken Bone Broth (page 53), and Vegetable Broth (page 52) throughout the duration of the meal plan. One recipe yields eight servings, so you can make them on the weekend to have ready for the entire week.

Beware that week 1 might be the time when you are most likely to give up on the plan due to so-called die-off effects, which can have you not feeling your best. Die-off occurs when bacteria or yeast die off and the body releases pro-inflammatory proteins in response to an influx of toxins. Die-off can cause irritability, fatigue, (even more) digestive issues, headaches, brain fog, and other flu-like symptoms. But keep in mind that these symptoms are temporary—and could be an indicator that you are on the right path.

It is completely normal to feel discouraged when you start to feel these effects, but you must remember that after the rain comes the rainbow! If the die-off effects feel extreme, consider these strategies for managing them:

- activated charcoal supplements (for reducing the body's inflammatory responses to toxins)

- glutathione supplements (the body's master antioxidant)

- increased water intake

- sleep

- infrared sauna treatments

- Epsom salt baths

- exercise (as tolerated, to move waste through the lymphatic system)

Even if you're not suffering from die-off effects, throughout the 4-week plan, you should focus heavily on drinking more water. The benefits of staying hydrated for digestion are endless. The health of every cell and synapse depends on it. And when you're even a little dehydrated on a regular basis, your metabolism, energy, and immunity all suffer mightily.

Here are three reasons drinking lots of water is critical for digestion—and even more so if you have gut healing to do:

1. Water helps combat fatigue, headaches, hunger, and sugar cravings. All of those can lead to digestive problems and stress.

2. Water helps move the digestive system along. If you are constipated, lack of water could be the cause.

3. Water helps eliminate toxins from the body via sweat, urine, and feces. Toxins cause irritation and inflammation, damaging the gut even more.

If you drink a cup or two of hot water with lemon or lime per day, your digestive system will benefit even more. Lemons and limes are alkaline-forming, and since disease does not thrive in an alkaline environment, your gut will benefit. Lemons and limes also help purify the liver by liquefying bile while inhibiting excess bile flow.

For some people, it may be the case that drinking liquids with meals inhibits proper digestion. Your best option then is to drink water, tea, and straight broth in between meals rather than with food.

Week 1 is likely to be the week when the most change is being made, and any change in life can be difficult. But nothing changes if nothing changes, so get ready for a real change to start taking place!

WEEK 1 SHOPPING LIST

CANNED AND BOTTLED ITEMS

❑ Pumpkin purée, 1 (29-ounce) can

❑ Salmon, 1 (14¾-ounce) can

❑ Tuna, albacore in water,
  3 (5-ounce) cans

DAIRY AND EGGS

❑ Eggs, large (4)

❑ Milk, almond (or non-soy plant-based
  milk of choice), unsweetened (½ gallon)

FROZEN FOODS

❑ Blueberries, 1 (12-ounce) bag

❑ Cauliflower, 2 (12-ounce) bags

❑ Spinach, 1 (8-ounce) bag

❑ Strawberries, 1 (12-ounce) bag

MEAT AND FISH

❑ Beef, bones (1 pound)

❑ Chicken, bones (1 pound)

❑ Chicken, drumsticks (18)

❑ Chicken, whole (4 pounds)

❑ Pork, 4 (6-ounce) boneless chops

❑ Pork, loin (1 pound)

❑ Salmon, 4 (4-ounce) fillets

❑ Scallops, large (1 pound)

❑ Turkey, ground (1 pound)

PANTRY ITEMS

❑ Cinnamon, ground

❑ Dill, dried

❑ Flaxseed, ground

❑ Flour, coconut

❑ Garlic powder

❑ Gelatin, unflavored

❑ Hemp seeds

❑ Maple syrup

❑ Mustard, Dijon

❑ Oil, coconut

❑ Oil, olive

❑ Oregano, dried

❑ Peppercorns, black

❑ Salt

❑ Stevia or monk fruit

❑ Tea bags, caffeine-free

❑ Turmeric, ground

❑ Vanilla extract

❑ Vinegar, apple cider

❑ Vinegar, red-wine

PRODUCE

❑ Apple (1)

❑ Avocado (1)

❑ Bananas (3)

❑ Bay leaves, 1 (¾-ounce) package

❑ Basil, 1 bunch

❑ Blueberries (2 pints)

❑ Brussels sprouts, 1 (8-ounce) bag

❑ Carrots, baby, 1 (12-ounce) bag

❑ Carrots, whole (9) plus 1 pound

❑ Celery (1 bunch)

❑ Cilantro (2 bunches)

❑ Dill, 1 (¾-ounce) package

❑ Garlic (2 heads)

- ❏ Ginger (1 small piece)
- ❏ Kale (1 bunch)
- ❏ Leeks (2)
- ❏ Lemons (8)
- ❏ Onions, red (2)
- ❏ Onions, yellow (6)
- ❏ Parsley, flat-leaf (2 bunches)
- ❏ Peaches (4)
- ❏ Rosemary, 2 (¾-ounce) packages
- ❏ Sage, 1 (¾-ounce) package
- ❏ Spinach, baby, 2 (10-ounce) packages
- ❏ Sweet potatoes (2)
- ❏ Swiss chard (1 bunch)
- ❏ Thyme, 2 (¾-ounce) packages

WEEK 1 MEAL PLAN

SUNDAY

BREAKFAST: On-the-Go Turkey Breakfast Muffins (page 70) with a cup of Vegetable Broth (page 52)

LUNCH: Salmon Patties (page 111)

DINNER: Sage and Thyme Roasted Chicken and Vegetables (page 97) with a cup of Chicken Bone Broth (page 53)

MONDAY

BREAKFAST: Blueberry Smoothie Bowl (page 74)

LUNCH: leftover Sage and Thyme Roasted Chicken and Vegetables (page 97) with a cup of Chicken Bone Broth (page 53)

DINNER: Lemon and Dill Broiled Salmon (page 106) with a cup of Vegetable Broth (page 52)

TUESDAY

BREAKFAST: Blueberry Gel (page 62) with leftover On-the-Go Turkey Breakfast Muffins (page 70)

LUNCH: leftover Salmon Patties (page 111)

DINNER: Baked Lemon-Pepper Chicken Drummies (page 96) with a cup of Beef Bone Broth (page 54)

WEDNESDAY

BREAKFAST: Strawberry-Vanilla Smoothie (page 73)

LUNCH: leftover Baked Lemon-Pepper Chicken Drummies (page 96) with a cup of Vegetable Broth (page 52)

DINNER: Red-Wine Vinegar-Glazed Pork Chops with Peaches (page 124)

THURSDAY

BREAKFAST: leftover On-the-Go Turkey Breakfast Muffins (page 70) with a cup of Beef Bone Broth (page 54)

LUNCH: leftover Red-Wine Vinegar-Glazed Pork Chops with Peaches (page 124)

DINNER: Pumpkin-Apple Soup (page 80)

FRIDAY

BREAKFAST: Boosted Green Smoothie (page 72)

LUNCH: leftover Pumpkin-Apple Soup (page 80)

DINNER: Lemon-Pepper Tuna (page 104)

SATURDAY

BREAKFAST: Blueberry Smoothie Bowl (page 74)

LUNCH: leftover Lemon-Pepper Tuna (page 104) with a cup of Chicken Bone Broth (page 53)

DINNER: Creamy Spinach Soup (page 83)

WEEK 2: REPLACE

Now that we have removed the foods that have potentially been contributing to your leaky gut, in week 2 it's time to replace them with foods that will support your gut healing.

Every bit of food we consume makes its way through the digestive system, which means that it is imperative that we have the necessary digestive secretions to process that food. In this phase, we will begin replacing the digestive secretions that may have been previously missing with enzymes, bile salts, and hydrochloric acid.

Enzymes are required in the body for everything from reducing inflammation to proper hormone regulation, energy production, fighting infections, and healing wounds. They help break down food into smaller parts that can be absorbed, transported, and utilized by every cell in the body.

The body produces less of these enzymes as we age, so ensuring we have enough is critical for healing leaky gut syndrome. By age 40, your enzyme production could be 25 percent lower than it was when you were a child. Here are some signs that you might be producing low levels of digestive enzymes: bloating, diarrhea, constipation, floating stools, weak nails, rashes, dull skin, hair thinning or loss, fatigue, headaches, insomnia, flatulence, malabsorption, and mood swings.

We can supplement with digestive enzymes or begin increasing enzyme levels naturally through eating more raw, living foods like fermented vegetables and raw honey and chewing all foods thoroughly. Some foods that naturally contain digestive enzymes include pineapple, papaya, mango, honey, banana, cultured yogurt, avocado, kefir, sauerkraut, kimchi, miso, kiwi, and ginger.

Bile is a digestive liquid that's produced in the liver to help break down fats and allow the body to excrete cholesterol and potentially toxic compounds. Bile salts help facilitate this process. Among other things, having sufficient bile helps fight off infection, promotes gallbladder and liver function, and allows for fats and nutrients to be absorbed. Insufficient bile can lead to vitamin deficiencies (namely A, D, E, and K), heartburn, bloating and other digestive issues (trapped gas, diarrhea, bad-smelling gas, stomach cramps), gallstones, hormonal imbalance, low cholesterol levels, and liver damage.

In addition to supplementing with bile salts, those with low levels of bile should stay very hydrated and consume beets and beet greens (a powerful liver detoxifier). They should also increase the number of different fruits and vegetables they eat to give the body a vast array of nutrients, eat more healthy fats (like omega-3s), and consume more calcium (though not from high-fat dairy).

Finally, hydrochloric acid (HCl) is critical for gut health because it breaks down food for digestion. HCl, like digestive enzymes, decreases as we age. Hypochlorhydria is a condition in which the body doesn't produce enough stomach acid in order to break down proteins into essential amino acids and nutrients the body needs. Some signs that you have low stomach acid include diarrhea, gas, SIBO, bloating, difficulty digesting meat, undigested food in stools, acne and eczema, and a vitamin B12 deficiency.

In conjunction with a doctor or other medical professional, you can do a simple at-home stomach acid test. You will need to ingest betaine HCl (preferably with pepsin) along with a higher-protein meal.

If you discover that you have low stomach acid, here are some ways you can naturally increase it: add fermented vegetables, high-quality sea salt, ginger, dandelion root, lemon, and apple cider vinegar to your diet; marinate your meats; and chew thoroughly.

In addition to replacing some of these digestive secretions during week 2, we will still continue eating in the same way as in week 1 in order to reset the body.

During week 2, some people already start feeling better. If you're still not feeling your best, though, don't worry. This is also completely normal, and many people require at least three full weeks before they can detect any sort of light at the end of the tunnel.

As you wrap up week 2, you can start looking forward to the second half of the 4-week leaky gut diet meal plan, along with the fact that you're about to embark on even more healing. Trust the process!

WEEK 2 SHOPPING LIST

Note: From weeks 2 to 4, you may not need to make more Beef Bone Broth (page 54), Chicken Bone Broth (page 53), or Vegetable Broth (page 52). Monitor the amount you have left, and when you start running low, prepare a new batch. In order to do this, you will need to include those ingredients *in addition to* the ingredients on the shopping list below.

CANNED AND BOTTLED ITEMS

❑ Milk, coconut, full-fat, 5 (13½-ounce) cans

❑ Milk, coconut, light, 2 (13½-ounce) cans

❑ Pineapple, diced, 1 (20-ounce) can

DAIRY AND EGGS

❑ Eggs, large (14)

❑ Milk, almond (or non-soy plant-based milk of choice), unsweetened (½ gallon)

MEAT AND FISH

❑ Beef, ground (3 pounds)

❑ Beef, lean stew meat (1¼ pounds)

❑ Chicken, boneless, skinless breasts or thighs (1 pound)

❑ Pork or turkey, sausage, bulk (1 pound)

❑ Shrimp, baby, cooked, 1 (16-ounce) bag

❑ Shrimp, medium, cooked, 1 (12-ounce) bag

❑ Tilapia, 4 (6-ounce) fillets

❑ Turkey breasts, boneless (3 pounds)

PANTRY ITEMS

❑ Allspice, ground

❑ Baking soda

❑ Cardamom

❑ Chia seeds

❑ Cinnamon, ground

❑ Coconut aminos

❑ Flour, coconut

❑ Garlic powder

❑ Gelatin, unflavored

❑ Ginger, ground

❑ Hemp seeds

❑ Honey

❑ Maple syrup

❑ Miso paste

❑ Mustard, Dijon

❑ Nutmeg, ground

❑ Oil, coconut

❑ Oil, olive

❑ Oregano, dried

❑ Pecans, raw

❑ Peppercorns, black

❑ Peppermint extract, pure

❑ Poultry seasoning

❑ Salt

- ❑ Sesame seeds
- ❑ Sugar, coconut
- ❑ Turmeric, ground
- ❑ Vanilla extract
- ❑ Vinegar, apple cider

PRODUCE

- ❑ Arugula, 1 (8-ounce) bag
- ❑ Asparagus (1 bunch)
- ❑ Avocados (6)
- ❑ Beet (1)
- ❑ Blueberries (2 pints)
- ❑ Broccoli florets, 4 (12-ounce) bags
- ❑ Cabbage, Napa (1 head)
- ❑ Cabbage, purple (1 head)
- ❑ Carrots, whole, 2 (1-pound) bags
- ❑ Celery (1 bunch)
- ❑ Cilantro (1 bunch)
- ❑ Cucumbers (5)
- ❑ Dill (1 bunch)
- ❑ Garlic (1 head)
- ❑ Ginger (1 large piece)
- ❑ Kale (1 bunch)
- ❑ Lemons (9)
- ❑ Lettuce, butter (1 head)
- ❑ Lettuce, romaine (2 heads)
- ❑ Limes (5)
- ❑ Mango (1)
- ❑ Mint (2 bunches)
- ❑ Onion, red (1)
- ❑ Onion, yellow (1)
- ❑ Parsley (1 bunch)
- ❑ Papaya (1)
- ❑ Peppers, bell, red (2)
- ❑ Plantains, ripe (4)
- ❑ Scallions (1 bunch)
- ❑ Spinach, 1 (10-ounce) bag
- ❑ Squash, butternut (2)
- ❑ Squash, yellow (summer) (6)
- ❑ Strawberries (1 pound)
- ❑ Sweet potato, large (1)
- ❑ Tomato (1)
- ❑ Swiss chard (1 bunch)
- ❑ Thyme (1 bunch)
- ❑ Zucchini (1)

OTHER

- ❑ Probiotics (60 capsules)

WEEK 2 MEAL PLAN

SUNDAY

BREAKFAST: Eggs and Greens Buddha Bowl (page 71)

LUNCH: Fermented Veggies (page 60) with leftover Creamy Spinach Soup (page 83)

DINNER: Chicken Lettuce Wraps with Creamy Honey-Lemon Dressing (page 93) with a cup of Beef Bone Broth (page 54)

MONDAY

BREAKFAST: Coconut Yogurt (page 57) with blueberries (if desired)

LUNCH: leftover Chicken Lettuce Wraps with Creamy Honey-Lemon Dressing (page 93) with a cup of Vegetable Broth (page 52)

DINNER: leftover Fermented Veggies (page 60) with Honey-Ginger-Garlic Beef Stir-Fry (page 116)

TUESDAY

BREAKFAST: Strawberry-Vanilla Smoothie (page 73)

LUNCH: leftover Honey-Ginger-Garlic Beef Stir-Fry (page 116)

DINNER: Baked Garlic Chicken Drummies (page 92)

WEDNESDAY

BREAKFAST: leftover Coconut Yogurt (page 57)

LUNCH: leftover Baked Garlic Chicken Drummies (page 92)

DINNER: Swedish Meatballs (page 118) with a cup of Vegetable Broth (page 52)

THURSDAY

BREAKFAST: Mango-Mint Chia Pudding (page 76)

LUNCH: Everyday Tossed Salad with Apple Cider Vinaigrette (page 89)

DINNER: Ginger-Coconut Butternut Bisque (page 81)

FRIDAY

BREAKFAST: Boosted Green Smoothie (page 72)

LUNCH: leftover Swedish Meatballs (page 118)

DINNER: Baked Tilapia with Creamy Cilantro Sauce (page 108) with a cup of Beef Bone Broth (page 54)

SATURDAY

BREAKFAST: Autoimmune Paleo Bread (sweet version; page 56)

LUNCH: leftover Ginger-Coconut Butternut Bisque (page 81)

DINNER: Summer Paleo Shrimp Succotash (page 107) with a cup of Vegetable Broth (page 52)

WEEK 3: REPAIR

The goal of week 3 is to continue building on the work we did during week 1 (removing) and week 2 (replacing) and really begin repairing the gut lining and soothing any remaining inflammation.

We will focus on repairing the gut lining by adding some soothing (and critical) nutrients such as antioxidants, omega-3 fatty acids, turmeric, and glutamine. In addition, probiotic and prebiotic foods will become a mainstay so that the beneficial bacteria can begin to repopulate.

All along, we have been incorporating broths and soups into our diet. You have likely been consuming more (and different) broth and soups than ever before in your life. This is very intentional. Remember, bone broth (and high-quality stock in general) has a multitude of benefits that will take gut-restoring potential to the next level.

Another key nutrient we will stock up on more during week 3 is antioxidants. Some of the foods containing antioxidants we will consume this week include blueberries, kale, purple cabbage, spinach, cinnamon, walnuts, and turmeric. Turmeric is a top detoxifying agent and has been known to soothe inflammation while assisting with leaky gut syndrome healing. Turmeric dramatically increases the antioxidant capacity of the body by protecting it from free radicals.

We will also focus this week on omega-3 fatty acids. Studies have consistently shown a connection between higher omega-3 intake and reduced inflammation. Reducing inflammation is soothing, and this is part of our goal during week 3 (and throughout the 4-week meal plan as a whole).

Two foods that are high in omega-3 fatty acids are salmon and walnuts, both of which you'll enjoy this week. Salmon is also a great source of protein and B vitamins (which are often lacking in those with leaky gut syndrome). Walnuts are a super source of plant-based omega-3 fatty acids; they help promote a healthy gut in general by decreasing overall inflammation and supporting weight control.

Finally, week 3 has the option for including or increasing the amount of glutamine (another anti-inflammatory) in your meals. Glutamine helps prevent and repair leaky gut, heals inflammation, and boosts the overall immune system.

You can get glutamine from certain foods, such as bone broth, grass-fed beef, asparagus, wild-caught fish like cod and salmon, and turkey. Some find it easier, though, to supplement with L-glutamine capsules or powder. The powder is odorless and mostly tasteless, so adding it to your bowls, soups, broths, puddings, smoothies, and juices is a very quick and easy way to incorporate it into your everyday diet.

During week 3, you might very well feel the best you have since starting. If not, something to consider trying is meal spacing. Meal spacing is used for optimal digestion to allow the migrating motor complex to complete its cleansing wave. It is a cyclic, recurring motility pattern that occurs in the stomach and small bowel during fasting; it is interrupted by feeding. You can practice meal spacing by waiting to eat until at least 3 hours since you last ate, since the cleansing wave occurs every 90 to 120 minutes while fasting. As a bonus, when the digestive system is given a break, the body is not processing anything, so there is nothing to feed any unwanted bacteria.

WEEK 3 SHOPPING LIST

DAIRY AND EGGS

- ❑ Eggs, large (8)
- ❑ Ghee (8 ounces)
- ❑ Milk, almond (or non-soy plant-based milk of choice), unsweetened (½ gallon)
- ❑ Milk, coconut, full-fat, 2 (13½-ounce) cans
- ❑ Milk, walnut (8 ounces)

MEAT AND FISH

- ❑ Bacon, 1 (16-ounce) package
- ❑ Beef, ground (1 pound)
- ❑ Chicken, boneless, skinless breasts or thighs (1 pound)
- ❑ Cod, 4 (4-ounce) fillets
- ❑ Pork, ground (1 pound)
- ❑ Salmon, 4 (4-ounce) fillets
- ❑ Salmon, wild, 2 (6-ounce) fillets
- ❑ Turkey, ground (2 pounds)

PANTRY ITEMS

- ❑ Almond extract
- ❑ Baking soda
- ❑ Cardamom, ground
- ❑ Chia seeds
- ❑ Cinnamon, ground
- ❑ Cocoa powder, unsweetened
- ❑ Coconut aminos
- ❑ Cumin, ground
- ❑ Curry powder
- ❑ Hemp seeds

- ❑ Flaxseeds
- ❑ Flour, coconut or almond
- ❑ Garlic powder
- ❑ Ginger, ground
- ❑ Hazelnuts, raw
- ❑ Honey
- ❑ Macadamia nuts
- ❑ Maple syrup
- ❑ Oil, coconut
- ❑ Oil, olive
- ❑ Olives, Kalamata, pitted (8 ounces)
- ❑ Peppercorns, black
- ❑ Salt
- ❑ Sesame seeds
- ❑ Stevia
- ❑ Sugar, coconut
- ❑ Turmeric, ground
- ❑ Vanilla extract
- ❑ Vinegar, apple cider
- ❑ Vinegar, white balsamic
- ❑ Walnuts, raw

PRODUCE

- ❑ Arugula, 1 (6-ounce) bag
- ❑ Bananas, green (2)
- ❑ Bananas, yellow (2)
- ❑ Basil (2 bunches)
- ❑ Blackberries (1 pint)
- ❑ Broccoli florets, 1 (12-ounce) bag
- ❑ Brussels sprouts (8 ounces)
- ❑ Cabbage, purple (1 head)

- ❑ Capers (2½ Tablespoons)
- ❑ Carrot (1)
- ❑ Cauliflower, head (1)
- ❑ Celery, stalks (3)
- ❑ Cherries, pitted (8 ounces)
- ❑ Cilantro (1 bunch)
- ❑ Cucumbers (1) plus 4 Persian cucumbers
- ❑ Dill (1 bunch)
- ❑ Garlic (1 head)
- ❑ Ginger (1 piece)
- ❑ Green beans (¼ cup)
- ❑ Kale (1 bunch)
- ❑ Lemons (2)
- ❑ Lemongrass (1 small bunch)
- ❑ Marjoram (1 bunch)
- ❑ Mushrooms, sliced, 2 (8-ounce) packages
- ❑ Onion, red (1)
- ❑ Onion, white (1)
- ❑ Parsley, flat-leaf (1 bunch)
- ❑ Peppers, bell, green (1)
- ❑ Peppers, bell, red (1)
- ❑ Sage, 1 bunch
- ❑ Scallions (1 bunch)
- ❑ Spinach, 2 (10-ounce) bags
- ❑ Spring mix, 1 (5-ounce) bag
- ❑ Squash, spaghetti (1)
- ❑ Sweet potatoes (4)
- ❑ Tomatoes, cherry, 2 (10-ounce) cartons

WEEK 3 MEAL PLAN

SUNDAY

BREAKFAST: Soothing Golden Latte (page 58)

LUNCH: Cucumber and Blueberry Summer Salad with Blueberry Vinaigrette (page 86)

DINNER: Guilt-Free Turkey Burgers (page 98)

MONDAY

BREAKFAST: leftover Autoimmune Paleo Bread (sweet version) (page 56)

LUNCH: leftover Summer Paleo Shrimp Succotash (page 107)

DINNER: Lemongrass Chicken Curry (page 94) with a cup of Chicken Bone Broth (page 53)

TUESDAY

BREAKFAST: Blueberry Smoothie Bowl (page 74)

LUNCH: leftover Guilt-Free Turkey Burgers (page 98)

DINNER: Wild Salmon Salad with Blackberry Vinaigrette (page 84)

WEDNESDAY

BREAKFAST: Plantain Breakfast Muffins (page 67)

LUNCH: leftover Lemongrass Chicken Curry (page 94)

DINNER: Lemon and Dill Broiled Salmon (page 106) with a cup of Vegetable Broth (page 52)

THURSDAY

BREAKFAST: Strawberry-Vanilla Smoothie (page 73)

LUNCH: leftover Lemon and Dill Broiled Salmon (page 106)

DINNER: Honey-Garlic Baked Cod (page 110) and a cup of Chicken Bone Broth (page 53)

FRIDAY

BREAKFAST: Eggs and Greens Buddha Bowl (page 71)

LUNCH: leftover Honey-Garlic Baked Cod (page 110)

DINNER: Pork Stir-Fry with Purple Cabbage (page 122)

SATURDAY

BREAKFAST: Bacon, Eggs, and Crispy Brussels Sprouts (page 68)

LUNCH: leftover Pork Stir-Fry with Purple Cabbage (page 122) with a cup of Beef Bone Broth (page 54)

DINNER: One-Pan Turmeric Beef and Broccoli (page 123)

WEEK 4: REBALANCE

The goal of week 4 is to rebalance the gut microbiome by continuing on with the diet changes begun in the previous three weeks, but we'll be heavily focusing on the lifestyle component as well.

The diet portion won't change much, except that the goal for rebalancing is to encourage even more good bacteria to populate. This is done through the use of prebiotic and probiotic foods, and many people choose to incorporate a probiotic supplement as well.

During week 4, you'll likely be eating a wider variety of foods than during the first three weeks of the plan. As you're adding a few more things in, take note of how your body is responding. Is it positive? Negative? Not sure yet? If you listen closely to it, your body is *always* telling you something. Adjust as necessary.

But diet isn't the only thing to focus on this week. One key principle for healing leaky gut is that you absolutely must address four main lifestyle elements: stress management, sleep habits, exercise, and stimulation of the vagus nerve.

1. **STRESS MANAGEMENT.**
   The importance of managing stress all boils down to the connection between the gut and the brain. Indeed, the enteric nervous system, which is the part of the nervous system that governs the GI tract, has been described as a "second brain." When we talk about stress, it's not just the familiar too-much-on-my-plate kind of stress. Instead, it's separated into five main categories: physical stress, environmental stress, biological stress, sociological stress, and psychological stress. All of this stress can cause or worsen leaky gut syndrome. There are many different approaches to managing stress; start with the ones listed under "stimulation of the vagus nerve" below.

2. **SLEEP HABITS.**
   Poor sleep habits translate to poor gut health. Insufficient or low-quality sleep leads to increased overall body inflammation, which compromises proper gut functioning. The National Sleep Foundation says that adults need at least seven hours of sleep per night, and those with a compromised immune system or leaky gut syndrome could need even more.

3. **EXERCISE.**

   Getting the right amount of the right kind of exercise is an important lifestyle factor for overcoming leaky gut syndrome. Too little physical activity may weaken the digestive system, but too much activity has been shown to negatively impact the immune system. During gut-healing periods, it's important to consider both the intensity and duration of any exercise. A workout should leave you feeling energized rather than drained; it should be fun and not a stressful burden. When you finish exercising, your stomach should feel fine—you shouldn't feel bloated and need to rush to the bathroom immediately.

4. **STIMULATION OF THE VAGUS NERVE.**

   The vagus nerve, the longest of the cranial nerves, controls the parasympathetic nervous system, which can be thought of as your inner nerve center. The parasympathetic nervous system is sometimes called the "rest and digest" system because it increases intestinal activity and relaxes the sphincter muscles in the GI tract. It is also highly involved in preventing inflammation, initiating the body's relaxation response, and communicating between the gut and brain. Stress, anxiety, alcohol, improper nutrition, overworking, and lack of sleep prevent the vagus nerve from doing its job, leading to inflammation, leaky gut syndrome, and more. Here are five things that will help stimulate the vagus nerve this week and until you're healed: deep breathing exercises, light exercise, a probiotic-rich diet, yoga or meditation, and splashing your face with cold water.

If you can give it your all for this final week, especially as it relates to the lifestyle pieces, this can be the week when you'll really begin feeling the positive effects of the 4-week program.

WEEK 4 SHOPPING LIST

CANNED AND BOTTLED ITEMS

- ❑ Mandarin oranges, 1 (15-ounce) can
- ❑ Milk, coconut, full-fat, 1 (13½-ounce) can
- ❑ Milk, coconut, light (8 ounces)
- ❑ Olives, black, sliced, 2 (6-ounce) cans
- ❑ Tomato sauce, no salt added, 1 (8-ounce) can
- ❑ Tuna, albacore, 2 (5-ounce) cans

DAIRY AND EGGS

- ❑ Eggs, large (8)
- ❑ Goat cheese, 2 (4-ounce) packages

FROZEN FOODS

- ❑ Peas, 1 (10-ounce) bag

MEAT AND FISH

- ❑ Bacon (8 ounces)
- ❑ Beef, ground (4¼ pounds)
- ❑ Chicken, bone-in, skin-on thighs (4)
- ❑ Turkey, sausage, bulk (1 pound)

PANTRY ITEMS

- ❑ Almond meal
- ❑ Almonds
- ❑ Baking soda
- ❑ Coconut aminos
- ❑ Cinnamon, ground
- ❑ Cumin, ground
- ❑ Flaxseed, ground
- ❑ Flour, coconut

- ❑ Garlic powder
- ❑ Hemp seeds
- ❑ Honey
- ❑ Maple syrup
- ❑ Oil, coconut
- ❑ Oil, olive
- ❑ Oregano, dried
- ❑ Paprika
- ❑ Peppercorns, black
- ❑ Pumpkin pie spice
- ❑ Salt
- ❑ Sesame seeds
- ❑ Sugar, coconut
- ❑ Vinegar, apple cider
- ❑ Vinegar, white balsamic
- ❑ Walnuts
- ❑ Yeast, nutritional

PRODUCE

- ❑ Apples, green (1)
- ❑ Arugula (1 bunch)
- ❑ Avocados (1)
- ❑ Bananas (3)
- ❑ Basil (1 bunch)
- ❑ Brussels sprouts (4 cups)
- ❑ Celery (1 bunch)
- ❑ Cilantro (1 bunch)
- ❑ Garlic (1 head)
- ❑ Grapes, red (2 cups)
- ❑ Lemons (2)
- ❑ Limes (1)
- ❑ Mint (1 bunch)

- ❑ Onions, red (2)
- ❑ Onion, yellow (2)
- ❑ Parsley, flat-leaf (1 bunch)
- ❑ Peppers, bell, red (2)
- ❑ Rosemary (1 bunch)
- ❑ Sage (1 bunch)
- ❑ Scallions (1 bunch)
- ❑ Shallots (2)
- ❑ Snow peas (½ pound)
- ❑ Spinach, baby, 1 (5-ounce) package
- ❑ Spring mix, 1 (8-ounce) bag

- ❑ Squash, spaghetti (1)
- ❑ Squash, yellow (summer) (1)
- ❑ Sweet potatoes (5)
- ❑ Thyme (1 bunch)
- ❑ Tomato, Roma (1)
- ❑ Tomatoes, cherry (1 pint)
- ❑ Zucchini (1)

OTHER

- ❑ Probiotics (60 capsules)

WEEK 4 MEAL PLAN

SUNDAY

BREAKFAST: Spring Pea Omelet with Goat Cheese (page 66)

LUNCH: leftover One-Pan Turmeric Beef and Broccoli (page 123)

DINNER: Turkey and Sweet Potato Casserole (page 101)

MONDAY

BREAKFAST: Perfect Vegan Banana Spoon Bread (page 75)

LUNCH: leftover Turkey and Sweet Potato Casserole (page 101)

DINNER: One-Pan Maple-Garlic Chicken and Sweet Potatoes (page 95)

TUESDAY

BREAKFAST: Coconut Yogurt (page 57) with leftover Perfect Vegan Banana Spoon Bread (page 75)

LUNCH: leftover One-Pan Maple-Garlic Chicken and Sweet Potatoes (page 95)

DINNER: Beef Burgers with Browned Shallots (page 117)

WEDNESDAY

BREAKFAST: Blueberry Smoothie Bowl (page 74)

LUNCH: leftover Beef Burgers with Browned Shallots (page 117)

DINNER: Kitchen Sink Vegetable Sauté (page 135)

THURSDAY

BREAKFAST: Eggs and Greens Buddha Bowl (page 71) with leftover Coconut Yogurt (page 57)

LUNCH: leftover Kitchen Sink Vegetable Sauté (page 135)

DINNER: Skillet Turkey Sausage and Sweet Potatoes (page 99) with a cup of Chicken Bone Broth (page 53)

FRIDAY

BREAKFAST: Boosted Green Smoothie (page 72)

LUNCH: leftover Skillet Turkey Sausage and Sweet Potatoes (page 99)

DINNER: Tomato and Basil No-Dough Pizza (page 119)

SATURDAY

BREAKFAST: Spring Pea Omelet with Goat Cheese (page 66)

LUNCH: Vegetable Chowder (page 82) with Fermented Veggies (page 60)

DINNER: Mini Beef and Bacon Meatballs (page 121)

BEYOND THE 4 WEEKS

What good is a 4-week leaky gut syndrome meal plan if you go back to the old ways on day one of the fifth week? If you revert to your old diet and lifestyle, some or all of your previous symptoms will likely come back—and you may even experience some new ones.

To begin the next phase of your healing journey, consider writing down where you've been, where you are now, and where you want to go. Be aware of the things you'll have to do in order to get there.

Then, begin by reintroducing even more foods if you are ready for it. If you're feeling good, you can consider fermented or sprouted grains, soaked legumes, and other gut-friendly dairy like grass-fed butter and organic yogurt. You might also choose to start adding other pseudograins, like quinoa.

Be sure to proceed slowly and carefully. If you reintroduce everything on day one and you have immediate symptoms, you won't know exactly what triggered them. Add one new thing every two to four days to help explore your own body and digestive system's needs even more.

If you find yourself suffering from something you ate, don't beat yourself up over it. Remember, stress plays a huge role in your leaky gut syndrome healing. Let it go, and try again tomorrow to stay with the plan.

What if, after the four weeks are up, you still feel miserable, and adding even more foods is making you feel worse? The best recommendation is to simply scale back. Get back to the very basics of broth, soups, and other foods that tend to be easier to digest. You can stay there as long as you need to, but be sure to keep adding things in as you start feeling better. If you eat only the very basics for too long, new issues could arise.

No two people are the same, and no two digestive systems will act and react in the same way. For some, four weeks may not be enough time to see dramatic health changes, but if you have followed the meal plan and lifestyle recommendations and still haven't found relief, consider additional research and testing. As noted in chapter 1, leaky gut syndrome accompanies many other illnesses, diseases, and general conditions.

For example, if you have undiagnosed SIBO and you are following this meal plan to the letter, you may find yourself still bloated after eating otherwise gut-healthy foods like fermented veggies, garlic, onion, and kombucha. If you have undiagnosed diverticulitis, you may have a problem when eating too many nuts or seeds. And if you have any undiagnosed autoimmune condition, you might notice exacerbated symptoms when eating things like bell peppers and tomatoes.

The list of scenarios and situations is endless. And in these more severe cases, the best next step is to test, not guess. If you want to get on (or stay on) the gut-healing path, you'll first need to find out what else is contributing to or causing the leaky gut.

For many other people, though, these past four weeks will have been life-changing in the sense that all symptoms and issues have been resolved. If this is you, you are likely less bloated or have less diarrhea, your appetite has stabilized, your cravings have diminished, your skin is clearer, and your mind is sharper. The energy you have today is more than you've had in previous months combined. Maybe most important is the fact that you now feel like the *you* you've been waiting for to come back!

Keep sticking with the healthy diet and finding the right balance of all your life stressors. It will be your ultimate key to success.

PROBIOTICS AND PREBIOTICS

Probiotics and prebiotics often go hand in hand, but they are not the same thing. Probiotics are the good and beneficial bacteria we need for a healthy gut; prebiotics are the foods that feed that bacteria.

You can take a probiotic supplement or get probiotics from foods like cultured yogurt, kefir, miso, fermented sauerkraut, and kombucha. Prebiotics are commonly added to foods these days in the form of ingredients like inulin and chicory. But they are also found in whole-food sources like tomatoes, garlic, onions, and asparagus.

Now that you understand what they are and how they are used, it makes sense as to why they would be removed (or mostly removed) during week 1 of the plan. The reason is simply that not all probiotics and prebiotics are right for everyone at every stage along the healing journey. But the goal is to arrive at a place where you are consuming both probiotics and prebiotics, because our digestive system does thrive with the combination.

ONE-PAN MAPLE-GARLIC CHICKEN AND SWEET POTATOES, PAGE 95

....

PART TWO

The Recipes

All of the recipes in this section have been carefully considered for their leaky gut healing properties, but they are also nutritious and delicious. The goal is to make these next four weeks feel exciting because you'll be preparing and trying new dishes. Yes, even dessert!

Each recipe includes the number of servings, length of time to prep and cook, and appropriate week to introduce the dish. In addition, the recipes specify whether they are gluten-free, nut-free, dairy-free, or vegetarian or vegan, and also whether they can be made in under 30 minutes, can be made in one pot, or contain no more than five ingredients. Nutritional information is also included for each recipe.

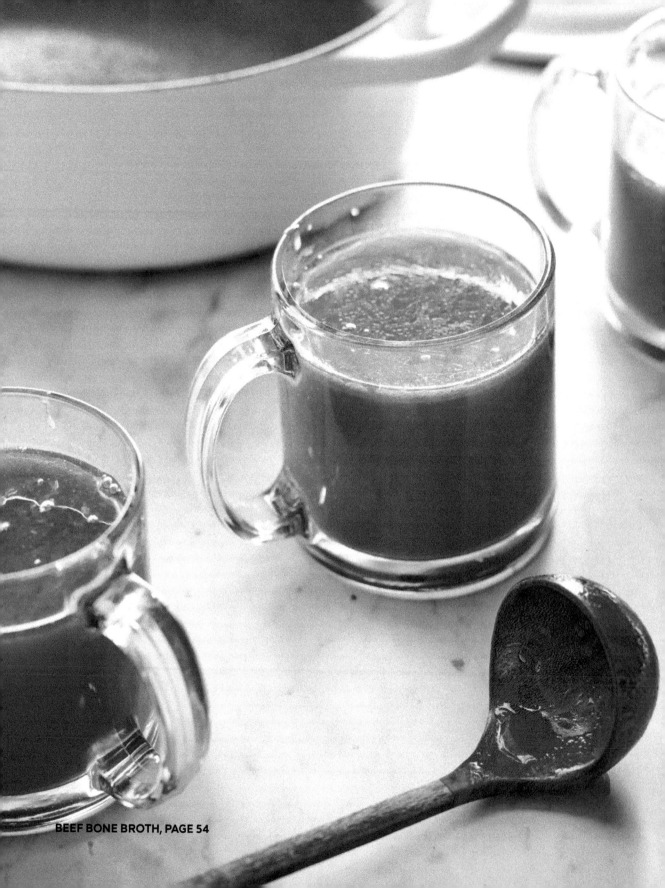

BEEF BONE BROTH, PAGE 54

Foundation Recipes

Vegetable Broth

GLUTEN-FREE, NUT-FREE, DAIRY-FREE, VEGAN, ONE-POT

SERVES 8 / PREP TIME: 10 MINUTES / COOK TIME: 4 HOURS **Week 1**

Broth is the foundation for many leaky-gut diet plans. While bone broths are known to be the staple, there is a place for vegetable broths as well. The ingredients in this recipe are filled with vitamins, minerals, and nutrients that are extracted in liquid form into the broth. Enjoy this broth by the cup or use it as a base for soups and sauces.

5 garlic cloves, unpeeled and chopped

5 carrots, unpeeled and chopped

5 celery stalks, chopped

2 bay leaves

1 yellow onion, unpeeled and chopped

1 sweet potato, unpeeled and chopped

½ leek, cut into thirds

½ bunch fresh flat-leaf parsley, chopped

½ bunch fresh cilantro, chopped

½ (¾-ounce) package fresh rosemary

14 cups water

1 teaspoon salt

1. Combine the garlic, carrots, celery, bay leaves, onion, sweet potato, leek, parsley, cilantro, rosemary, water, and salt in a large soup pot. Bring to a boil over medium-high heat, then reduce the heat to a simmer, cover, and cook for 4 hours.

2. Strain the broth into another pot or a storage container, and discard the solids. Season with salt.

Make ahead: If you have an 8-quart multi-cooker (such as an Instant Pot), you can really speed up this process. Combine all the ingredients in the pot, cover, and seal. Using the "Manual" function, cook on High for 30 minutes. Leave the broth to sit for 1½ to 2 hours. Strain the broth into another pot or a storage container, and discard the solids. Season with salt.

Per Serving: Calories: 20; Total Fat: 0g; Saturated Fat: 0g; Sodium: 311mg; Carbohydrates: 4g; Fiber: 1g; Protein: 0g

Chicken Bone Broth

GLUTEN-FREE, NUT-FREE, DAIRY-FREE, ONE-POT

SERVES 8 / PREP TIME: 10 MINUTES / COOK TIME: 4 HOURS Week 1

Enjoyed by the cup or as the base for soups and sauces, this chicken bone broth recipe will become a new household staple. Infused with lemon and several herbs, the flavor will have your taste buds bouncing and your gut healing like never before. For convenience, pour some of the broth into an ice cube tray to use any time a recipe calls for a small amount.

1 pound chicken bones (plus any leftover giblets from cooking whole chicken, if you have them)

2 carrots, unpeeled and cut into thirds (if you have the tops, use those, too)

2 garlic cloves, unpeeled and chopped

2 bay leaves

1 celery stalk, cut into thirds

1 lemon, halved

½ leek, cut into thirds

½ red onion, cut into thirds, unpeeled and chopped

½ yellow onion, cut into thirds, unpeeled and chopped

½ (¾-ounce) package fresh rosemary

½ (¾-ounce) package fresh thyme

½ bunch fresh cilantro, chopped

15 cups water

2 tablespoons apple cider vinegar

Salt

Freshly ground black pepper

1. Combine the chicken bones, carrots, garlic, bay leaves, celery, lemon, leek, red onion, yellow onion, rosemary, thyme, cilantro, water, vinegar, salt, and pepper in a large soup pot. Bring to a boil over medium-high heat, then reduce the heat to a simmer, cover, and cook for 4 hours.

2. Strain the broth into another pot or a storage container, and discard the solids. Season with salt.

Make ahead: If you have an 8-quart multi-cooker (such as an Instant Pot), you can really speed up this process. Combine all the ingredients in the pot, cover, and seal. Using the "Manual" function, cook on High for 30 minutes. Leave the broth to sit for 1½ to 2 hours. Strain the broth into another pot or a storage container, and discard the solids. Season with salt.

Per Serving: Calories: 24; Total Fat: 0g; Saturated Fat: 0g; Sodium: 340mg; Carbohydrates: 1g; Fiber: 0g; Protein: 4g

Beef Bone Broth

GLUTEN-FREE, NUT-FREE, DAIRY-FREE, ONE-POT

SERVES 8 / PREP TIME: 10 MINUTES / COOK TIME: 4 HOURS 15 MINUTES **Week 1**

Filled with flavor, this beef bone broth will satisfy your savory cravings while helping heal your gut. The key to the flavor-filled broth extracted from this recipe is that the bones are roasted first. A smoky, rich flavor will soothe the gut almost immediately.

1 pound beef bones

2 tablespoons olive oil

Salt

Freshly ground black pepper

3 bay leaves

2 garlic cloves, unpeeled and chopped

2 carrots, unpeeled and cut into thirds (if you have the tops, use those, too)

1 celery stalk, cut into thirds

½ leek, cut into thirds

½ red onion, unpeeled and chopped

½ yellow onion, unpeeled and chopped

½ bunch fresh flat-leaf parsley, chopped

½ bunch fresh cilantro, chopped

15 cups water

2 tablespoons apple cider vinegar

1. Preheat the oven to 425°F. Line a rimmed baking sheet with aluminum foil.
2. Put the bones on the prepared baking sheet. Brush with the oil, and season with a little salt and pepper.
3. Transfer the baking sheet to the oven, and bake until the bones have a gently roasted, golden color, for about 15 minutes. Remove from the oven.
4. Transfer the bones to a large soup pot.
5. Add the bay leaves, garlic, carrots, celery, leek, red onion, yellow onion, parsley, cilantro, water, and vinegar. Bring to a boil over medium-high heat, then reduce to a simmer, cover, and cook for 4 hours.
6. Strain the broth into another pot or a storage container, and discard the solids. Season with salt.

Did you know? Once the broth has cooled and been placed in the refrigerator, it should form a gelatinous layer on top. Don't throw it out! Instead, warm the broth in a small pan on the stove. The gelatin will melt, and you will be sure to reap all its gut-healing benefits.

Per Serving: Calories: 40; Total Fat: 1g; Saturated Fat: 1g; Sodium: 280mg; Carbohydrates: 5g; Fiber: 1g; Protein: 6g

Savory Turmeric Flatbread

GLUTEN-FREE, DAIRY-FREE, VEGAN, UNDER 30 MINUTES

SERVES 4 / PREP TIME: 10 MINUTES / COOK TIME: 20 MINUTES **Week 3**

This tasty flatbread is so versatile, you'll find many different ways to enjoy it. Eat it warm with a bit of coconut oil on top, use it to make a sandwich, or cut it up into strips to use as a salad topper. It contains nutrient-dense ingredients like hemp seeds, garlic, and turmeric. Turmeric can also contribute to healthy digestion, thanks to its antioxidant and anti-inflammatory properties.

2 medium green bananas, chopped

6 tablespoons water

2 tablespoons coconut oil, melted

2 tablespoons hemp seeds

1½ tablespoons coconut flour

1 tablespoon ground flaxseed

1 tablespoon chia seeds

1 teaspoon ground turmeric

1 teaspoon garlic powder

1 teaspoon salt

1. Preheat the oven to 400°F. Line a 9-by-13-inch baking dish with parchment paper.
2. In a blender, combine the bananas, water, oil, hemp seeds, flour, flaxseed, chia seeds, turmeric, garlic powder, and salt. Blend until smooth.
3. Pour the mixture into the prepared dish, and spread it out into a thin layer.
4. Transfer the dish to the oven, and bake until golden brown around the edges, for about 17 minutes. Remove from the oven.
5. Serve the flatbread warm, or let cool and store in an airtight container at room temperature for up to 2 days.

Per Serving: Calories: 215; Total Fat: 14g; Saturated Fat: 7g; Sodium: 538mg; Carbohydrates: 21g; Fiber: 6g; Protein: 5g

Autoimmune Paleo Bread

GLUTEN-FREE, DAIRY-FREE

SERVES 6 / PREP TIME: 10 MINUTES / COOK TIME: 20 TO 30 MINUTES **Week 2**

The best part about this recipe is that you can make either a sweet or a savory bread with the same ingredients. If you want a sweet bread, choose very ripe plantains; if you want a savory bread, choose very green plantains. Instead of eggs, this recipe uses gelatin, which is healing for the gut.

Olive oil, for brushing

2 large plantains, sliced

2 tablespoons coconut flour

2 teaspoons baking soda

1½ teaspoons ground cinnamon

1½ teaspoons ground ginger

14 tablespoons water, divided

3 tablespoons gelatin

1. Preheat the oven to 400°F. Brush a 9-inch round cake pan lightly with oil.
2. In a blender, combine the plantains, flour, baking soda, cinnamon, and ginger.
3. Put 7 tablespoons of water in a large jar with a lid.
4. Put the remaining 7 tablespoons of water in a small saucepan, and heat over medium heat until near boiling. Remove from the heat, and pour into the jar.
5. Add the gelatin, cover the jar tightly, and shake vigorously until the gelatin has completely dissolved, for about 1 minute.
6. Pour the gelatin mixture into the blender. Blend until smooth, and pour into the prepared cake pan.
7. Transfer the pan to the oven and bake until a toothpick inserted into the center comes out clean, for 20 to 23 minutes (for the savory bread version) or 27 to 30 minutes (for the sweet bread version). Remove from the oven.
8. Let the bread cool in the pan, then slice and enjoy.

Did you know? Autoimmune Paleo is one of the strictest gut-healing protocols used for autoimmune conditions. The protocol eliminates not only everything the leaky-gut diet does but also nightshades, nuts, seeds, added sugars, legumes, and eggs.

Per Serving: Calories: 114; Total Fat: 2g; Saturated Fat: 1g; Sodium: 354mg; Carbohydrates: 23g; Fiber: 4g; Protein: 5g

Coconut Yogurt

GLUTEN-FREE, DAIRY-FREE, VEGAN, ONE-POT, 5 INGREDIENTS OR LESS

SERVES 2 / PREP TIME: 5 MINUTES, PLUS AT LEAST 24 HOURS TO SET **Week 2**

Cultured yogurt is filled with beneficial probiotics. Using full-fat coconut milk to make this yogurt ensures that it is also dairy-free (as long as your probiotic is vegan). Enjoy it with a little raw honey or fresh fruit, or as a topper for pudding or Blueberry Gel (page 62). If you want a thicker yogurt, use less of the water in the coconut milk can; use more (or all of it) for a thinner yogurt.

1 (13½-ounce) can full-fat coconut milk

2 probiotic capsules

1. Pour the coconut milk into a jar.
2. Using a wooden or ceramic spoon (do not use a metal spoon), stir the coconut milk until smooth.
3. Open the probiotic capsules, pour the powder into the jar, and stir it in with the same spoon.
4. Cover the jar with a piece of cheesecloth, and secure it with a rubber band.
5. Leave the jar on the counter but out of direct sunlight for 24 to 48 hours (depending on how warm your house is), tasting occasionally.
6. Once the yogurt has a tangy flavor, remove the cheesecloth, and cover the jar with a lid.
7. Put the yogurt in the refrigerator for a couple of hours to thicken and firm. Keep refrigerated, and consume within a couple of days.

Substitution tip: You can use organic dairy milk to make this yogurt, if desired.

Per Serving: Calories: 435; Total Fat: 45g; Saturated Fat: 40g; Sodium: 28mg; Carbohydrates: 11g; Fiber: 4g; Protein: 4g

Soothing Golden Latte

GLUTEN-FREE, DAIRY-FREE, VEGAN, UNDER 30 MINUTES, ONE-POT

SERVES 2 / PREP TIME: 5 MINUTES / COOK TIME: 5 MINUTES **Week 2**

I predict this beverage will soon become a staple in your household. The warming, healing spices of turmeric, ginger, cardamom, and cinnamon make this a great way to start or end the day. It's good on a cold or warm day and can instantly bring about a calm mood.

2 cups unsweetened almond milk (or non-soy plant-based milk of choice)

1 tablespoon coconut sugar

1 teaspoon ground turmeric

1 teaspoon ground cinnamon

¼ teaspoon ground ginger

Pinch ground cardamom

1. In a small saucepan, heat the milk over medium heat until slightly warm, for about 5 minutes.
2. Add the sugar, turmeric, cinnamon, ginger, and cardamom, and stir with a whisk until combined. Remove from the heat, pour into mugs, and enjoy.

Substitution tip: If you prefer, you can replace the coconut sugar with stevia or monk fruit.

Per Serving: Calories: 114; Total Fat: 6g; Saturated Fat: 0g; Sodium: 231mg; Carbohydrates: 10g; Fiber: 3g; Protein: 3g

3-Ingredient Sauerkraut

GLUTEN-FREE, NUT-FREE, DAIRY-FREE, VEGAN, 5 INGREDIENTS OR LESS

SERVES 16 / PREP TIME: 10 MINUTES, PLUS AT LEAST 24 HOURS TO FERMENT Week 2

"Sauerkraut" is a German word that translates to "sour cabbage" in English. This recipe will yield a sour, tangy sauerkraut that pairs well with salty foods. Sauerkraut is helpful for rebuilding beneficial gut bacteria, so you might want to just eat a tablespoon on its own each day.

½ medium head Napa cabbage, shredded

1 tablespoon salt

Juice of 1 lemon

1. In a large bowl, combine the cabbage, salt, and lemon juice.
2. Knead the mixture with your hands until there is enough liquid to cover, for about 10 minutes.
3. Pack the cabbage into a 1-quart jar (or 2 smaller jars), pressing down on the cabbage so it is submerged in the liquid. If necessary, add a bit of water to completely cover the cabbage.
4. Cover the jar with a piece of cheesecloth, a paper towel, or a coffee filter; secure it with a rubber band.
5. Leave the sauerkraut to ferment on the counter. Start tasting it after 2 or 3 days. The aroma should be strong, sour, and vinegary but still pleasant. The vegetables should taste sour but not spoiled or rotten.
6. Once the desired level of fermentation has been reached, serve. Or cover the jar tightly and store in the refrigerator.

Did you know? Sauerkraut is made by a process called lacto-fermentation. The lacto-fermenting process gets rid of bad bacteria in the first stage, then lets the good bacteria go to work during the second stage.

Per Serving: Calories: 8; Total Fat: 0g; Saturated Fat: 0g; Sodium: 443mg; Carbohydrates: 1g; Fiber: 1g; Protein: 1g

Fermented Veggies

GLUTEN-FREE, NUT-FREE, DAIRY-FREE, VEGAN

SERVES 16 / PREP TIME: 15 MINUTES, PLUS AT LEAST 24 HOURS TO FERMENT **Week 2**

Fermented vegetables make for a flavorful, colorful addition to many meals. They're filled with probiotics and nutrients that are healing for the gut.

2 carrots, peeled and shredded or chopped

1 small beet, peeled and shredded or chopped

½ head Napa cabbage, shredded

½ head purple cabbage, shredded

Juice of 1 lime

4 cups water

2 tablespoons salt

1. In a large bowl, combine the carrots, beet, napa cabbage, purple cabbage, and lime juice, and mix well.

2. Transfer the mixture to a clean wide-mouth jar (or several smaller jars, if desired), leaving at least 1½ inches of headspace.

3. In a large liquid measuring cup or medium bowl, mix the water and salt until the salt has dissolved.

4. Pour the salt water brine over the vegetables in the jar, leaving 1 inch of headspace.

5. Cover the jar with a piece of cheesecloth, a paper towel, or a coffee filter; secure with a rubber band.

6. Leave the vegetables to ferment on the counter for 3 to 7 days, checking on them daily to make sure all the vegetables are staying below the brine. The vegetables will exude more liquid, but if you notice after 24 hours that the liquid does not cover all the vegetables, add some water and a pinch of salt.

7. Start tasting the vegetables after 2 or 3 days. The aroma should be strong, sour, and vinegary but still pleasant. The vegetables should taste sour but not spoiled or rotten.

8. Once the desired level of fermentation has been reached, serve. Or cover the jar tightly and store in the refrigerator.

Did you know? For best results when fermenting your own vegetables, ensure that the vegetables are all cut into similar sizes, always submerge the vegetables in liquid to keep them in an oxygen-free environment (otherwise mold will occur), and make certain that the jar(s) you use are extra clean.

Per Serving: Calories: 13; Total Fat: 0g; Saturated Fat: 0g; Sodium: 482mg; Carbohydrates: 3g; Fiber: 1g; Protein: 1g

Blueberry Gel

GLUTEN-FREE, NUT-FREE, DAIRY-FREE, ONE-POT, 5 INGREDIENTS OR LESS

SERVES 4 / PREP TIME: 10 MINUTES, PLUS 4 HOURS TO SET **Week 1**

Gelatin has known gut-healing benefits, but you won't need to buy Jell-O once you learn how easy it is to make your own. Blueberries give this gel a pleasant, fruity flavor, and they are also a powerful antioxidant, which contributes to overall reduced inflammation.

4 cups water, divided

3 tea bags, caffeine-free, any flavor

1¼ cups fresh blueberries, divided

2 tablespoons stevia or monk fruit

2 tablespoons gelatin

1. In a small saucepan, bring 3 cups of water to near-boiling.
2. Remove the pan from the heat, add the tea bags, and let them steep for 8 to 10 minutes.
3. In a blender, combine ½ cup of water, ¼ cup of blueberries, and the stevia. Blend until completely mixed together.
4. Pour the blueberry mixture into a medium bowl, add the remaining ½ cup of water, then very slowly whisk in the gelatin until dissolved.
5. Discard the tea bags. Add the tea to the blueberry mixture, and whisk until completely combined.
6. Pour the mixture into an 8-by-8-inch baking dish, then scatter the remaining 1 cup of blueberries on top. Cover and refrigerate until firm and set, for 4 to 5 hours.

Substitution tip: Consider using ginger, lavender, mint, or lemon balm tea, all of which have antioxidants and gut-healing properties.

Per Serving: Calories: 38; Total Fat: 0g; Saturated Fat: 0g; Sodium: 7mg; Carbohydrates: 8g; Fiber: 1g; Protein: 3g

EGGS AND GREENS BUDDHA BOWL, PAGE 71

CHAPTER FOUR

Breakfast

Spring Pea Omelet with Goat Cheese

GLUTEN-FREE, NUT-FREE, VEGETARIAN, UNDER 30 MINUTES, ONE-POT

SERVES 1 / PREP TIME: 5 MINUTES / COOK TIME: 10 MINUTES **Week 4**

Hearty and delicious, this omelet makes for a perfect weekend or weekday breakfast. Thanks to simple ingredients like eggs, goat cheese, and mint, it has a light, fresh flavor. Goat cheese is a natural probiotic and a good alternative to cow's milk cheese because it's lower in lactose.

2 large eggs

¼ cup frozen peas, thawed

1 scallion, green part only, sliced

1 teaspoon chopped fresh mint, plus more for garnish

1 tablespoon olive oil

4 teaspoons goat cheese

Salt

Freshly ground black pepper

1. In a bowl, whisk together the eggs, peas, scallion, and mint.
2. In a small skillet, heat the oil over medium heat.
3. Pour the egg mixture into the pan.
4. Cook until the egg mixture begins to set at the edges, for 1 to 2 minutes, then tilt the pan, and gently push the cooked portions from the edges toward the center so that the uncooked eggs can reach the hot pan surface. Continue cooking in this manner until there is almost no visible liquid egg left.
5. Drop in the goat cheese teaspoon by teaspoon.
6. Carefully fold the omelet in half with a spatula, and cook until the cheese has melted, for about 30 seconds.
7. Slide the omelet onto a plate. Season with salt and pepper, then garnish with more chopped mint.

Make ahead: This omelet reheats beautifully! You can make it and then refrigerate it in an airtight container for up to 2 days. When ready to eat, put the omelet in a small skillet on the stove, and heat over medium heat for about 3 minutes. Alternatively, you can heat it in the microwave for 30 to 45 seconds.

Per Serving: Calories: 317; Total Fat: 26g; Saturated Fat: 6g; Sodium: 318mg; Carbohydrates: 7g; Fiber: 2g; Protein: 16g

Plantain Breakfast Muffins

GLUTEN-FREE, DAIRY-FREE, VEGETARIAN, UNDER 30 MINUTES

SERVES 12 / PREP TIME: 5 MINUTES / COOK TIME: 25 MINUTES   Week 2

These muffins are intended for breakfast, but because they are naturally sweet—thanks to the ripened plantains—you'll feel as though you're eating dessert. Lemon juice, cinnamon, and ginger all contain healing and soothing components to start the day off right. If you like a little more sweetness, top your muffin with some local raw honey, which contains natural digestive enzymes.

2 large ripe plantains, thinly sliced

2 large eggs

2 large egg whites

Juice of 1 lemon

¼ cup coconut flour

2 tablespoons coconut oil, melted

1 tablespoon ground cinnamon

1 tablespoon vanilla extract

1½ teaspoons minced fresh ginger

½ teaspoon baking soda

1. Preheat the oven to 350°F. Line a standard muffin tin with cupcake liners.
2. In a blender, combine the plantains, eggs, egg whites, lemon juice, flour, oil, cinnamon, vanilla, ginger, and baking soda. Blend until smooth.
3. Fill each cup of the muffin tin about three-quarters full with batter.
4. Transfer the muffin tin to the oven, and bake until a toothpick inserted into the center comes out clean, for 22 to 25 minutes, keeping a close eye on them the last few minutes so they don't overcook. Remove from the oven, and let cool before serving.

Substitution tip: If you are unable to find plantains for this recipe, you can swap them out for regular bananas. Use one large extremely unripe (green) banana and one large ripe banana (yellow with brown spots).

Per Serving: Calories: 97; Total Fat: 4g; Saturated Fat: 3g; Sodium: 71mg; Carbohydrates: 14g; Fiber: 3g; Protein: 3g

Bacon, Eggs, and Crispy Brussels Sprouts

GLUTEN-FREE, DAIRY-FREE, UNDER 30 MINUTES

SERVES 2 / PREP TIME: 10 MINUTES / COOK TIME: 20 MINUTES **Week 3**

A spin-off of the traditional bacon and eggs, this meal includes added healing and flavor boosters like Brussels sprouts and sage. The meal has a savory flavor with various textures, including a crunch that comes from the hazelnuts. Sage contains antioxidants and compounds that can help relax the gut.

8 ounces Brussels sprouts, leaves only (about 18 Brussels sprouts)

1 tablespoon olive oil, divided

1 or 2 pinches salt

1 cup chopped bacon

½ cup raw hazelnuts, halved

2 large eggs

1 tablespoon chopped fresh sage

Freshly ground black pepper

1. Preheat the oven to 375°F.
2. Trim the Brussels sprouts, then put them in a large bowl. Invert another bowl over the top, and shake vigorously until all the leaves have fallen off.
3. Put all the leaves in one bowl, and toss them with ½ tablespoon of oil. Season with the salt.
4. Spread out the leaves in a single layer on a large rimmed baking sheet.
5. Transfer the baking sheet to the oven, and bake until the leaves are slightly crispy, for about 6 minutes. Remove from the oven.
6. Meanwhile, line a plate with a paper towel. Fry the bacon in a large skillet over medium-high heat until cooked through. Using a slotted spoon, transfer the bacon to the paper towel to drain.
7. Add the remaining ½ tablespoon of oil and the hazelnuts to the bacon fat in the pan. Cook over medium heat until browned, for about 5 minutes. Use the slotted spoon to transfer the hazelnuts to the plate with the bacon.
8. Finally, prepare the eggs to your liking.
9. To serve, make a bed of Brussels sprout leaves on a plate, add the bacon and hazelnuts, and top with the eggs. Season with the sage, salt, and pepper.

Substitution tip: If you don't like hazelnuts, feel free to substitute almonds, cashews, walnuts, or another nut you prefer. Or you can use a seed like sesame or hemp, in which case you don't need to sauté them.

Per Serving: Calories: 704; Total Fat: 57g; Saturated Fat: 12g; Sodium: 1493mg; Carbohydrates: 18g; Fiber: 8g; Protein: 36g

On-the-Go Turkey Breakfast Muffins

GLUTEN-FREE, NUT-FREE, DAIRY-FREE, ONE-POT

SERVES 12 / PREP TIME: 10 MINUTES / COOK TIME: 25 MINUTES **Week 1**

Not only will these savory muffins satisfy your morning hunger pangs, but also they are packed with ingredients known to aid in gut healing: garlic, turmeric, and oregano. You can take these with you for a late-morning breakfast or snack on them throughout the day.

1 pound ground turkey

1 celery stalk, finely chopped

½ medium red onion, finely chopped

2 tablespoons ground flaxseed

1 teaspoon ground turmeric

½ tablespoon garlic powder

½ teaspoon freshly ground black pepper

½ teaspoon salt

½ teaspoon dried oregano

1. Preheat the oven to 375°F. Line a standard muffin tin with cupcake liners.
2. In a large bowl, combine the turkey, celery, onion, flaxseed, turmeric, garlic powder, pepper, salt, and oregano. Using a fork, mix until evenly distributed.
3. Fill each cup of the muffin tin about three-quarters of the way with the mixture.
4. Transfer the muffin tin to the oven, and bake until lightly browned, for 22 to 25 minutes, keeping a close eye on them the last few minutes so they don't overcook. Remove from the oven.

Make ahead: These muffins are perfect for baking and then taking along in the days to come. Once the muffins have cooled a bit, transfer them to an airtight container, and store in the refrigerator. When you're ready to eat a muffin, serve cold, heat in the microwave, or break it up in pieces, adding to soups, salads, or sautéed vegetables.

Per Serving: Calories: 58; Total Fat: 2g; Saturated Fat: 0g; Sodium: 99mg; Carbohydrates: 1g; Fiber: 1g; Protein: 8g

Eggs and Greens Buddha Bowl

GLUTEN-FREE, NUT-FREE, DAIRY-FREE, UNDER 30 MINUTES, ONE-POT

SERVES 2 / PREP TIME: 5 MINUTES / COOK TIME: 20 MINUTES **Week 2**

Everyone loves big Buddha bowls because they allow for so many different flavors, textures, and nutrients in one bowl. This one is simple yet nutrient-dense, with an array of greens, olive oil, avocado, eggs, and seeds.

4 tablespoons olive oil, divided

1 pound ground pork or turkey sausage

2 large eggs, beaten

2 cups torn spinach leaves

2 cups torn arugula leaves

2 cups torn kale leaves

1 avocado, pitted, peeled, and sliced

Scallions, sliced, for garnish

Sesame seeds, for garnish

Salt

Freshly ground black pepper

1. In a large skillet, heat 1 tablespoon of oil over medium heat.
2. Add the sausage and cook, breaking up the meat with a wooden spoon, until cooked through, for 5 to 7 minutes. Transfer the sausage to a bowl.
3. In the same pan, heat 1 tablespoon of oil over medium heat.
4. Add the eggs, and scramble them until cooked to your liking. Transfer to the bowl with the sausage.
5. In the same pan, heat the remaining 2 tablespoons of oil over medium heat.
6. Add the spinach, arugula, and kale, and sauté until wilted, for 3 to 5 minutes.
7. Build each bowl by placing the greens on the bottom, followed by the sausage, and finally, the eggs. Add avocado, scallions, and sesame seeds to taste, and season with salt and pepper.

Did you know? The traditional Buddha bowl is vegetarian. This one uses meat, but if you'd like to keep it traditional, simply remove the meat and add extra greens, avocado, and sesame seeds. And of course, you can prepare the eggs any way you like, such as over easy.

Per Serving: Calories: 917; Total Fat: 79g; Saturated Fat: 21g; Sodium: 1472mg; Carbohydrates: 22g; Fiber: 8g; Protein: 39g

Boosted Green Smoothie

GLUTEN-FREE, DAIRY-FREE, VEGAN, UNDER 30 MINUTES, ONE-POT

SERVES 1 / PREP TIME: 1 MINUTE Week 1

This smoothie is packed with nutrition and flavor while remaining low in sugar—the only sugar is found naturally, in the banana. Try this smoothie first thing in the morning for your boost of daily greens, with the confidence that it won't leave you drained from a sugar crash a few hours later.

1 cup unsweetened almond milk (or non-soy plant-based milk of choice)

2 tablespoons hemp seeds

1 teaspoon ground cinnamon

1 large handful kale

1 large handful spinach

1 banana, frozen

½ avocado

In a blender, combine the almond milk, hemp seeds, cinnamon, kale, spinach, banana, and avocado. Blend until smooth.

Did you know? Smoothies are a great way to pack in the nutrients and gut-healing foods like herbs, spices, and other boosts. Whenever desired, you can add other great gut-healing ingredients, such as L-glutamine, collagen, gelatin, quercetin, moringa, and ginger.

Per Serving: Calories: 531; Total Fat: 30g; Saturated Fat: 3g; Sodium: 350mg; Carbohydrates: 55g; Fiber: 16g; Protein: 17g

Strawberry-Vanilla Smoothie

GLUTEN-FREE, DAIRY-FREE, VEGAN, UNDER 30 MINUTES, ONE-POT, 5 INGREDIENTS OR LESS

SERVES 1 / PREP TIME: 1 MINUTE **Week 1**

This smoothie uses frozen cauliflower instead of a banana for thickening. If you've never tried this swap, you're in for a pleasant surprise, as cauliflower helps make the shake thick and creamy while adding a boost of fiber, vitamin C, magnesium, and potassium. The smoothie is lightly sweetened with strawberries and just a hint of maple syrup for a dessert-like treat first thing in the morning.

1½ cups unsweetened almond milk (or non-soy plant-based milk of choice)

1½ cups frozen strawberries

1½ cups frozen cauliflower florets

1 tablespoon vanilla extract

1 tablespoon maple syrup

In a blender, combine the almond milk, strawberries, cauliflower, vanilla, and maple syrup. Blend until smooth.

Substitution tip: You can use sweetened almond milk, if desired. When choosing a plant-based milk, be sure to read the ingredients. Avoid milks that have carrageenan, gums, and oils like rapeseed oil. Look for milks that contain five or fewer ingredients.

Per Serving: Calories: 262; Total Fat: 6g; Saturated Fat: 1g; Sodium: 318mg; Carbohydrates: 46g; Fiber: 10g; Protein: 5g

Blueberry Smoothie Bowl

GLUTEN-FREE, DAIRY-FREE, VEGAN, UNDER 30 MINUTES, ONE-POT

SERVES 2 / PREP TIME: 1 MINUTE **Week 1**

A smoothie bowl has the consistency of ice cream, making gut-healing breakfasts fun! This smoothie bowl uses a banana and blueberries to give it a hint of natural sweetness. The sweetness is evened out by adding in two vegetables, cauliflower and spinach. The combination of all these elements makes for a smoothie bowl worth eating daily.

2 cups unsweetened almond milk (or non-soy plant-based milk of choice)

1 cup frozen cauliflower florets

1 large banana, frozen

1 cup frozen spinach

1 cup frozen blueberries

½ cup fresh blueberries

1. In a blender, combine the almond milk, cauliflower, banana, spinach, and frozen blueberries. Blend until smooth.
2. Pour mixture into a bowl. Top with the fresh blueberries.

Substitution tip: Other gut-friendly toppings you could choose from include unsweetened shredded coconut, sliced bananas or other fresh fruits, and your favorite nuts and seeds.

Per Serving: Calories: 221; Total Fat: 7g; Saturated Fat: 0g; Sodium: 389mg; Carbohydrates: 36g; Fiber: 9g; Protein: 5g

Perfect Vegan Banana Spoon Bread

GLUTEN-FREE, DAIRY-FREE, VEGAN, ONE-POT

SERVES 4 / PREP TIME: 10 MINUTES / COOK TIME: 1 HOUR 5 MINUTES **Week 4**

This recipe is a take on traditional spoon bread, which is a moist cornmeal dish with a consistency more like pudding than bread. My version uses no eggs and just a bit of coconut flour, so the finished product has an even creamier texture than the original.

Coconut oil or olive oil, for brushing

2 medium ripe bananas

6 tablespoons water

2 tablespoons ground flaxseed

2 tablespoons maple syrup (optional)

⅓ cup coconut flour

1½ teaspoons ground cinnamon

1 teaspoon pumpkin pie spice

⅛ teaspoon salt

1 tablespoon apple cider vinegar

1 teaspoon baking soda

1. Preheat the oven to 350°F. Brush a 9-by-4-inch loaf pan with oil.
2. In a small bowl, combine the bananas, water, flaxseed, and maple syrup (if using). Mash and mix together.
3. In another bowl, whisk together the coconut flour, cinnamon, pumpkin pie spice, and salt.
4. Add the dry mixture to the wet, then add the vinegar and baking soda. Stir until completely combined, but do not overmix.
5. Pour the batter into the prepared pan.
6. Transfer the pan to the oven, and bake until the top is brown, for 60 to 65 minutes. Remove from the oven, and let cool before serving.

Did you know? Traditional baking powder contains corn, which is a top allergen, so people with leaky gut syndrome should avoid it. You can replace baking powder in most baked goods using a combination of apple cider vinegar and baking soda. Once the apple cider vinegar hits the baking soda, watch as it bubbles. This is the chemical reaction you want to see for effectiveness.

Per Serving: Calories: 197; Total Fat: 6g; Saturated Fat: 3g; Sodium: 351mg; Carbohydrates: 32g; Fiber: 13g; Protein: 5g

Mango-Mint Chia Pudding

GLUTEN-FREE, DAIRY-FREE, VEGAN, ONE-POT

SERVES 4 / PREP TIME: 5 MINUTES, PLUS 4 HOURS TO SET **Week 2**

Chia pudding is easy to make and can be enjoyed for breakfast, snack, and dessert. Mango makes a perfect fruity match for fresh mint. Peppermint is known to be soothing to the gut and can help with nausea as well. The chia seeds are packed with fiber to help move things through your digestive system.

1 (13½-ounce) can full-fat coconut milk

2 tablespoons maple syrup

¾ teaspoon pure peppermint extract

½ cup chia seeds

1½ cups diced fresh (or frozen and thawed) mango

Fresh mint, for garnish (optional)

1. In a large bowl, whisk together the coconut milk, maple syrup, and peppermint.
2. Whisk in the chia seeds.
3. Stir in the mango.
4. Cover the bowl (or divide the mixture into 4 mason jars and cover them) and refrigerate until set, for 4 to 5 hours.

Make ahead: You can make this chia pudding in the evening so it sets overnight.

Per Serving: Calories: 400; Total Fat: 31g; Saturated Fat: 21g; Sodium: 20mg; Carbohydrates: 31g; Fiber: 11g; Protein: 7g

MANDARIN ORANGE SALAD, PAGE 85

CHAPTER FIVE

Soups and Salads

Pumpkin-Apple Soup

GLUTEN-FREE, NUT-FREE, DAIRY-FREE, VEGAN

SERVES 4 / PREP TIME: 10 MINUTES / COOK TIME: 30 MINUTES **Week 1**

Not only for the Thanksgiving table, this soup can be served year-round. Full of sweet and savory flavors, it will leave you fully satisfied. Without even knowing it, you'll be getting the gut-healing benefits of broth since it's the liquid base to the soup.

1 tablespoon olive oil

1 small yellow onion, minced

1 teaspoon grated fresh ginger

3 cups pumpkin purée (from a 29-ounce can)

1 small apple, peeled if desired, then chopped

3 cups Vegetable Broth (page 52) or Chicken Bone Broth (page 53)

1 teaspoon ground cinnamon, plus more for serving

Salt

Freshly ground black pepper

1. In a large saucepan, heat the oil over medium heat.
2. Add the onion and ginger, and cook until browned, for about 3 minutes.
3. Add the pumpkin purée and apple, and cook until the apple has slightly softened, for 2 to 3 minutes.
4. Pour in the broth. Cover, reduce the heat, and simmer until the pumpkin and apple are soft, for about 20 minutes.
5. Remove the pan from the heat, and add the cinnamon.
6. Once the soup has cooled a bit, transfer to a blender, and process until smooth. (Alternatively, you can use an immersion blender to purée the soup right in the pan.)
7. Ladle into bowls, and top with more cinnamon, if desired.

Substitution tip: If you prefer a creamier soup, simply swap out the broth for your plant-based milk of choice. For the ultimate creaminess, use full-fat coconut milk.

Per Serving: Calories: 143; Total Fat: 4g; Saturated Fat: 1g; Sodium: 102mg; Carbohydrates: 26g; Fiber: 7g; Protein: 4g

Ginger-Coconut Butternut Bisque

GLUTEN-FREE, DAIRY-FREE, VEGAN

SERVES 4 / PREP TIME: 10 MINUTES / COOK TIME: 2 HOURS **Week 2**

Perfectly sweet and spicy, this soup tastes great and is naturally good for the gut. The main ingredient, butternut squash, is one of the most common varieties of winter squash. It offers a good supply of vitamin A, potassium, and fiber. With added ingredients like coconut oil, ginger, coconut milk, and soft carrot, the soup is both nutrient-dense and digestion-friendly.

1 medium butternut squash

1 tablespoon coconut oil

2 teaspoons grated fresh ginger

1 carrot, chopped

1 (13½-ounce) can light coconut milk

½ cup full-fat coconut milk

2½ tablespoons coconut sugar

Salt

Freshly ground black pepper

1. Preheat the oven to 350°F.
2. Cut the squash in half lengthwise. Place cut-side down in a 9-by-13-inch baking dish, and pour in about ¼ inch of water.
3. Transfer the dish to the oven, and bake until the squash has softened, for about 1½ hours. Remove from the oven.
4. Let the squash cool, then remove the skin and seeds. Transfer 5 cups of the flesh to a large bowl.
5. In a large saucepan, heat the oil over medium-low heat.
6. Add the ginger, and sauté until tender, for about 2 minutes.
7. Add the 5 cups of squash, the carrot, light coconut milk, full-fat coconut milk, and coconut sugar. Season with salt and pepper.
8. Increase the heat to a gentle boil, then reduce the heat to a simmer, cover, and cook until the carrot has softened, for about 20 minutes.
9. Using an immersion blender, blend into a thick, creamy soup. (Alternatively, you can use a potato masher for a chunkier texture.)

Make ahead: This soup can be divided into single-serving portions and stored in the freezer. When you're ready to consume, simply thaw and reheat over medium-low heat.

Per Serving: Calories: 266; Total Fat: 16g; Saturated Fat: 14g; Sodium: 85mg; Carbohydrates: 35g; Fiber: 5g; Protein: 4g

Vegetable Chowder

GLUTEN-FREE, DAIRY-FREE, VEGAN, UNDER 30 MINUTES, ONE-POT

SERVES 4 / PREP TIME: 5 MINUTES / COOK TIME: 25 MINUTES **Week 3**

This creamy vegan chowder swaps out potatoes with sweet potatoes, dairy milk with plant-based milk, and olive oil with butter. The vegetables, both sweet and savory, simmered in a savory broth, make for a complete meal. This chowder is also full of fiber, which helps move waste through the digestive system.

¼ cup olive oil

3 celery stalks, chopped

2 scallions, white and green parts, chopped

1 sweet potato, peeled and diced

1 carrot, chopped

½ cup green beans

1½ cups cherry tomatoes

1 teaspoon salt

¼ teaspoon freshly ground black pepper

2 cups unsweetened almond milk (or non-soy plant-based milk of choice)

1. In a large saucepan, heat the oil over medium-low heat.
2. Add the celery, scallions, sweet potato, carrot, and green beans, and cook until softened, for 10 minutes.
3. Add the tomatoes, salt, and pepper, and cook until the tomatoes are tender, for about 10 minutes.
4. Stir in the almond milk, and simmer until slightly thickened, for 3 minutes.

Substitution tip: To make this a heartier soup, add a can of wild salmon along with the almond milk.

Per Serving: Calories: 205; Total Fat: 16g; Saturated Fat: 2g; Sodium: 805mg; Carbohydrates: 14g; Fiber: 4g; Protein: 3g

Creamy Spinach Soup

GLUTEN-FREE, DAIRY-FREE, VEGAN, UNDER 30 MINUTES, ONE-POT

SERVES 4 / PREP TIME: 5 MINUTES Week 1

Perfect on a spring or summer day (or nestled in somewhere warm during fall and winter!), this light, cool soup will have you feeling extremely refreshed. Using minimal ingredients and plenty of lemon for soothing the gut, this recipe could become a gut-healing staple.

1 (10-ounce) bag fresh spinach

1 small yellow onion, chopped

2 cups unsweetened almond milk (or non-soy plant-based milk of choice)

2 tablespoons lemon juice

1½ tablespoons dried dill

Salt

Freshly ground black pepper

1. In a blender, combine the spinach, onion, almond milk, lemon juice, and dill. Blend until smooth.
2. Pour the mixture into a bowl, and season with salt and pepper.

Substitution tip: If you like trying new plant-based milks, this soup is great with either hazelnut or cashew milk. If you prefer a thicker soup, choose full-fat coconut milk.

Per Serving: Calories: 48; Total Fat: 2g; Saturated Fat: 0g; Sodium: 189mg; Carbohydrates: 6g; Fiber: 3g; Protein: 3g

Wild Salmon Salad with Blackberry Vinaigrette

GLUTEN-FREE, DAIRY-FREE, UNDER 30 MINUTES

SERVES 2 / PREP TIME: 10 MINUTES / COOK TIME: 10 MINUTES **Week 3**

This salad tastes great but is also highly anti-inflammatory. Both salmon and walnuts are high in omega-3 fatty acids. The blackberries are high in vitamin C, which helps combat inflammation and fight illness.

For the vinaigrette

1 cup fresh (or frozen and thawed) blackberries

½ cup olive oil

2 tablespoons white balsamic vinegar

1 tablespoon honey

Salt

For the salad

2 (6-ounce) wild salmon fillets

2 teaspoons coconut oil

Salt

2 cups spring salad mix

2 cups fresh spinach

½ cup raw walnuts, halved

Freshly ground black pepper

To make the vinaigrette

1. Preheat the oven to broil.
2. Meanwhile, in a blender, combine the blackberries, oil, vinegar, honey, and salt. Blend until smooth.

To make the salad

1. Place the salmon fillets on a small rimmed baking sheet. Top each with 1 teaspoon of coconut oil, and season with salt.
2. Transfer the baking sheet to the oven, and broil until the salmon has browned on top and cooked through, for 7 to 9 minutes. Remove from the oven.
3. Meanwhile, in a large bowl, toss together the salad mix, spinach, and walnuts.
4. Add the vinaigrette, and toss to coat.
5. Divide the salad between 2 plates.
6. Place a salmon fillet on top of each salad.

Substitution tip: If you don't have access to fresh salmon, you can replace it with 2 cans of wild salmon. Simply drain the salmon and add it to your salad.

Per Serving: Calories: 966; Total Fat: 80g; Saturated Fat: 15g; Sodium: 417mg; Carbohydrates: 22g; Fiber: 7g; Protein: 46g

Mandarin Orange Salad

GLUTEN-FREE, DAIRY-FREE, VEGAN, UNDER 30 MINUTES, ONE-POT

SERVES 3 / PREP TIME: 5 MINUTES **Week 4**

Here's a sweet citrus salad that is likely to pique your taste buds' interest. The crunchiness of celery and raw almonds creates a texture you'll love. Like all members of the citrus family, mandarin oranges provide a boost of vitamins and minerals that help support the immune system during your leaky-gut healing.

For the dressing

¼ cup olive oil

2 tablespoons coconut sugar

2 tablespoons white balsamic vinegar

½ teaspoon salt

Pinch freshly ground black pepper

For the salad

1 (5-ounce) bag baby spinach

2 scallions, chopped

1 (15-ounce) can mandarin oranges, drained

2 celery stalks, sliced

1 tablespoon minced fresh flat-leaf parsley

½ cup slivered raw almonds

To make the dressing

In a blender, combine the oil, sugar, vinegar, salt, and pepper. Blend until smooth.

To make the salad

1. In a large bowl, combine the spinach, scallions, oranges, celery, parsley, and almonds.
2. Pour the dressing over the salad, and toss to coat.

Substitution tip: You can swap out the 2 tablespoons coconut sugar in the dressing for 1 to 1½ tablespoons stevia or monk fruit, if desired.

Per Serving: Calories: 347; Total Fat: 26g; Saturated Fat: 3g; Sodium: 444mg; Carbohydrates: 29g; Fiber: 5g; Protein: 7g

Cucumber and Blueberry Summer Salad with Blueberry Vinaigrette

GLUTEN-FREE, NUT-FREE, DAIRY-FREE, VEGAN, UNDER 30 MINUTES, ONE-POT

SERVES 4 / PREP TIME: 10 MINUTES Week 2

There is nothing more refreshing in a salad than the combination of cucumbers and blueberries. This salad not only combines the two of them but also features a blueberry vinaigrette, which is a flavor boost. Finally, the salad uses fresh mint, which has been used for thousands of years to aid with upset stomachs or indigestion.

For the dressing

1 cup blueberries

½ cup olive oil

2 tablespoons white balsamic vinegar

1 tablespoon stevia

Salt

For the salad

5 cups peeled and diced cucumber (about 2 large cucumbers)

½ cup blueberries

1 tablespoon chopped fresh mint, plus more for garnish

1 teaspoon chopped fresh dill

To make the dressing

In a blender, combine the blueberries, oil, vinegar, and stevia. Season with salt. Blend until smooth.

To make the salad

1. In a large bowl, combine the cucumber, blueberries, mint, and dill.
2. Pour the dressing over the salad, and toss to coat. Garnish with mint.

Substitution tip: Whenever stevia is called for in a recipe, you can substitute monk fruit. Stevia is more widely available at grocery stores, but it can cause bloating, nausea, and gas in some people. Monk fruit is generally regarded as easier on the gut. Monk fruit is 150 to 200 times sweeter than sugar, and stevia is 200 to 300 times sweeter, so you'll need a little more monk fruit than the amount of stevia called for. Wherever a sweetener is called for, use what works best for you.

Per Serving: Calories: 273; Total Fat: 26g; Saturated Fat: 4g; Sodium: 43mg; Carbohydrates: 14g; Fiber: 2g; Protein: 2g

Taco Salad with Creamy Honey-Lemon Dressing

GLUTEN-FREE, DAIRY-FREE, UNDER 30 MINUTES

SERVES 3 / PREP TIME: 10 MINUTES / COOK TIME: 15 MINUTES **Week 4**

This recipe features all the best parts of a taco salad but leaves out any ingredients that could be inflammatory to the gut. By using a spring salad mix, you'll get a variety of easier-to-digest greens that are packed with fiber and nutrients.

For the dressing

3 large egg yolks

Juice of 1 lemon

¼ cup full-fat coconut milk

2 tablespoons olive oil

1 tablespoon honey

¼ teaspoon salt

For the salad

2 tablespoons olive oil

1 pound ground beef

½ yellow onion, chopped

1 (8-ounce) container spring salad mix

2 cups cherry tomatoes, halved

1 (6-ounce) can sliced black olives, drained

¼ bunch fresh cilantro, chopped

1 avocado, peeled, pitted, and sliced or diced

1 scallion, chopped

Salt

Freshly ground black pepper

To make the dressing

In a blender, combine the egg yolks, lemon juice, coconut milk, oil, honey, and salt. Blend until smooth.

To make the salad

1. In a large skillet, heat the oil over medium heat.
2. Add the ground beef and onion, and cook, stirring to break up the meat, until fully cooked, for about 12 minutes. Line a plate with a paper towel. Using a slotted spoon, transfer the ground beef mixture to the paper towel to drain.
3. In a large bowl, combine the spring mix, tomatoes, olives, and cilantro.
4. Add the ground beef mixture.
5. Pour the dressing over the salad, and toss to coat.
6. Top with the avocado and scallion, and season with salt and pepper.

Substitution tip: For a heartier salad, use romaine lettuce instead of the spring mix.

Per Serving: Calories: 701; Total Fat: 54g; Saturated Fat: 15g; Sodium: 732mg; Carbohydrates: 25g; Fiber: 9g; Protein: 36g

Simple Greek Salad with Non-Dairy Tzatziki Sauce

GLUTEN-FREE, NUT-FREE, DAIRY-FREE, VEGAN, UNDER 30 MINUTES, ONE-POT

SERVES 4 / PREP TIME: 10 MINUTES **Week 3**

A spin-off of a classic Greek dish, this vegan salad is a great way to get an extra dose of vitamin C into your day to help your immune system. The tzatziki sauce will not only complement this salad but also works well as a sauce over beef, bison, and chicken.

For the sauce

1 cucumber, peeled, seeded, and chopped

2 garlic cloves, chopped

Juice of ½ lemon

1½ cups full-fat coconut milk

1 tablespoon chopped fresh dill

¼ teaspoon salt

¼ teaspoon freshly ground black pepper

For the salad

1 (10-ounce) carton cherry tomatoes

1 green bell pepper, diced

1 red bell pepper, diced

4 Persian cucumbers, sliced

½ white onion, thinly sliced

2½ tablespoons capers

1 cup pitted kalamata olives

Freshly ground black pepper

To make the sauce

In a blender, combine the cucumber, garlic, lemon juice, coconut milk, dill, salt, and pepper. Blend until smooth.

To make the salad

1. In a medium bowl, combine the tomatoes, green bell pepper, red bell pepper, cucumbers, onion, capers, and olives. Season with pepper.

2. Pour the dressing over the salad, and toss to coat. Chill until ready to serve.

Did you know? Kalamata olives are rich in healthy fats and contain a natural antioxidant. If you can't find Kalamata olives in your grocery store, you can use black olives, which are slightly less briny.

Per Serving: Calories: 319; Total Fat: 26g; Saturated Fat: 20g; Sodium: 513mg; Carbohydrates: 24g; Fiber: 7g; Protein: 6g

Everyday Tossed Salad with Apple Cider Vinaigrette

GLUTEN-FREE, DAIRY-FREE, VEGETARIAN, UNDER 30 MINUTES, ONE-POT

SERVES 4 / PREP TIME: 10 MINUTES **Week 2**

This salad got its name because it's simple to toss together and uses ingredients that can be enjoyed every day. The dressing contains a boost of gut-healing properties from the apple cider vinegar, honey, and cinnamon.

For the dressing

6 tablespoons olive oil

1 tablespoon apple cider vinegar

1 tablespoon honey

1 teaspoon ground cinnamon

Salt

For the salad

1 carrot, shredded

½ red onion, sliced

4 cups chopped romaine lettuce

2 cups chopped Swiss chard

2 cups sliced strawberries

1 cup chopped purple cabbage

½ cup raw pecans, halved

To make the dressing

In a blender, combine the oil, vinegar, honey, and cinnamon. Season with salt. Blend until smooth. (Alternatively, you can whisk the ingredients together in a bowl.)

To make the salad

1. In a medium bowl, combine the carrot, onion, lettuce, chard, strawberries, cabbage, and pecans.
2. Pour the dressing over the salad, and toss to coat.

Substitution tip: If you don't like pecans, you can substitute cashews or walnuts, or simply omit them.

Per Serving: Calories: 342; Total Fat: 31g; Saturated Fat: 4g; Sodium: 96mg; Carbohydrates: 18g; Fiber: 5g; Protein: 3g

CHICKEN LETTUCE WRAPS WITH CREAMY
HONEY-LEMON DRESSING, PAGE 93

CHAPTER SIX

Poultry Mains

Baked Garlic Chicken Drummies

GLUTEN-FREE, NUT-FREE, DAIRY-FREE

SERVES 4 / PREP TIME: 5 MINUTES, PLUS 2 HOURS TO MARINATE / COOK TIME: 40 MINUTES **Week 1**

The oregano, garlic, and lemon in this marinade are all known to have healing properties for the gut. The flavors are simple yet powerful, and the chicken pairs nicely with greens marinated with olive oil and fresh lemon.

2 tablespoons olive oil

2 tablespoons lemon juice

¼ cup chopped fresh basil

2½ tablespoons dried oregano

2 teaspoons garlic powder

2 garlic cloves, minced

8 bone-in, skin-on chicken drumsticks

Salt

Freshly ground black pepper

1. In a large zip-top bag, combine the oil, lemon juice, basil, oregano, garlic powder, and garlic. Add the chicken, seal the bag, and toss to coat the chicken with the mixture.
2. Put the bag in the refrigerator, and marinate for at least 2 hours, turning the bag once or twice.
3. Preheat the oven to 400°F.
4. Remove the drumsticks from the bag, and arrange in a single layer on a rimmed baking sheet. Season with salt and pepper.
5. Transfer the baking sheet to the oven, and bake until the chicken is cooked through, for about 40 minutes. Remove from the oven.

Make ahead: Start marinating these drummies in the morning before you leave for work. Once you arrive home, preheat the oven—dinner will be ready in less than an hour!

Per Serving: Calories: 358; Total Fat: 21g; Saturated Fat: 5g; Sodium: 213mg; Carbohydrates: 4g; Fiber: 1g; Protein: 35g

Chicken Lettuce Wraps with Creamy Honey-Lemon Dressing

GLUTEN-FREE, DAIRY-FREE, UNDER 30 MINUTES

SERVES 4 / PREP TIME: 5 MINUTES / COOK TIME: 20 MINUTES **Week 2**

Using large romaine lettuce leaves instead of a bun is a simple swap for your gut-healing journey. These lettuce wraps are filled with flavor thanks to pineapple's natural sweetness. It has naturally occurring enzymes that help with the digestive process.

For the dressing

6 large egg yolks

Juice of 1 lemon

½ cup full-fat coconut milk

¼ cup olive oil

2 tablespoons honey

½ teaspoon salt

For the lettuce wraps

6 tablespoons olive oil, divided

1 (12-ounce) bag broccoli florets, chopped (about 4 cups)

2 cups chopped or shredded cooked chicken

1 (20-ounce) can pineapple, drained (about 2½ cups)

1 cup shredded carrot

Salt

Freshly ground black pepper

4 large romaine lettuce leaves

To make the dressing

In a blender, combine the egg yolks, lemon juice, coconut milk, oil, honey, and salt. Blend until smooth. (Alternatively, you can whisk the ingredients together in a bowl.)

To make the lettuce wraps

1. In a large wok or skillet, heat 3 tablespoons of oil over medium-high heat.
2. Add the broccoli and cook, stirring occasionally, until the broccoli has slightly browned, for about 10 minutes.
3. Add the remaining 3 tablespoons of oil, then the chicken, pineapple, and carrot. Season with salt and pepper.
4. Reduce the heat to medium, and cook until the pineapple is soft, 5 to 7 minutes. Remove from the heat.
5. Spread ⅓ to ½ cup of the mixture evenly onto each lettuce leaf. Drizzle with dressing, and roll up the wraps.

Substitution tip: You can easily make this a vegetarian dish by leaving out the chicken.

Per Serving: Calories: 704; Total Fat: 52g; Saturated Fat: 14g; Sodium: 402mg; Carbohydrates: 40g; Fiber: 6g; Protein: 29g

Lemongrass Chicken Curry

GLUTEN-FREE, NUT-FREE, DAIRY-FREE, UNDER 30 MINUTES, ONE-POT

SERVES 4 / PREP TIME: 10 MINUTES / COOK TIME: 15 MINUTES **Week 3**

This chicken dish has the beautiful flavor of lemongrass combined with a bit of heat from curry powder. The flavors are nicely balanced and provide a lot of gut-healing benefits. Lemongrass has traditionally been known to aid in digestion, and curry powder contains turmeric, which is an anti-inflammatory.

2 tablespoons coconut oil

½ red onion, thinly sliced

¼ cup finely chopped lemongrass (tender inner stalks only)

1 pound boneless, skinless chicken breasts or thighs, cut into bite-size pieces

½ teaspoon curry powder

Salt

Freshly ground black pepper

1. In a wok or large skillet, heat the oil over medium heat.
2. Add the onion and cook until browned, for about 3 minutes.
3. Add the lemongrass and cook, stirring, until fragrant, for 30 seconds.
4. Add the chicken and curry powder and cook, stirring, until the chicken has cooked through, about 10 minutes.
5. Taste and add more curry powder if desired, then season with salt and pepper.

Did you know? The finer you chop the lemongrass, the more flavor you'll extract. If you don't use the whole stalk, you can store any leftovers in an airtight container in the freezer.

Per Serving: Calories: 185; Total Fat: 8g; Saturated Fat: 6g; Sodium: 114mg; Carbohydrates: 1g; Fiber: 0g; Protein: 26g

One-Pan Maple-Garlic Chicken and Sweet Potatoes

GLUTEN-FREE, DAIRY-FREE, ONE-POT

SERVES 2 / PREP TIME: 10 MINUTES / COOK TIME: 50 MINUTES **Week 4**

This recipe requires just one pan, and although the ingredients are minimal, the finished dish includes many different flavors and textures. Maple syrup gives it a slight sweetness, and natural sugar is regarded as a great substitute for refined sugar during intense periods of gut healing.

2 tablespoons olive oil, divided

1 tablespoon coconut aminos

1 teaspoon maple syrup

2 garlic cloves, minced

1 large sweet potato, diced

4 bone-in, skin-on chicken thighs

3 rosemary sprigs

½ cup snow peas, ends trimmed

Salt

Freshly ground black pepper

1. Preheat the oven to 350°F.
2. In a medium bowl, whisk together 1 tablespoon of oil, the coconut aminos, maple syrup, and garlic.
3. Add the sweet potato, and toss to coat.
4. In a large cast iron skillet or other oven-safe pan, heat the remaining 1 tablespoon of oil over medium heat.
5. Add the chicken thighs and cook until browned, for 3 minutes on each side.
6. Add the sweet potato mixture and simmer until the sweet potato starts to soften, for 4 minutes.
7. Place the rosemary sprigs on top and transfer the pan to the oven. Bake for 20 minutes.
8. Add the snow peas, return the pan to the oven, and bake until the chicken has cooked through, about 20 minutes. Remove from the oven. Season with salt and pepper.

Substitution tip: Coconut aminos are a salty, savory seasoning sauce made from the fermented sap of coconut palm and sea salt. It has a milder, sweeter flavor than traditional soy sauce and is commonly found near the soy sauce in the grocery store. If you cannot find it, use tamari soy sauce, which is generally wheat-free (check the labeling to make sure).

Per Serving: Calories: 363; Total Fat: 24g; Saturated Fat: 5g; Sodium: 372mg; Carbohydrates: 21g; Fiber: 3g; Protein: 18g

Baked Lemon-Pepper Chicken Drummies

GLUTEN-FREE, NUT-FREE, DAIRY-FREE

SERVES 5 / PREP TIME: 5 MINUTES / COOK TIME: 45 MINUTES **Week 1**

Not only is this recipe filled with flavor, but also it's super easy to make. Lemon, pepper, and parsley are the main flavors; they provide a bit of tang and a bit of spice to the chicken for a tasty meal.

10 bone-in, skin-on chicken drumsticks

½ bunch fresh flat-leaf parsley, chopped

Grated zest and juice of 2 lemons

¼ cup olive oil

1½ teaspoons salt

1½ teaspoons freshly ground black pepper

1. Preheat the oven to 425°F.
2. Arrange the chicken drumsticks in a single layer in a 9-by-13-inch baking dish.
3. In a small bowl, whisk together the parsley, lemon zest and juice, oil, salt, and pepper. Pour over the chicken.
4. Transfer the dish to the oven and bake for 20 minutes.
5. Turn the drumsticks over, return the dish to the oven, and bake until cooked through, for 20 to 25 minutes.

Make ahead: To have dinner waiting for you when you get home from work, try making these in the slow cooker. Simply combine all the ingredients in the slow cooker, cover, and cook on Low for 5 to 6 hours.

Per Serving: Calories: 375; Total Fat: 24g; Saturated Fat: 6g; Sodium: 754mg; Carbohydrates: 1g; Fiber: 1g; Protein: 34g

Sage and Thyme Roasted Chicken and Vegetables

GLUTEN-FREE, DAIRY-FREE, ONE-POT

SERVES 4 / PREP TIME: 10 MINUTES / COOK TIME: 2 HOURS **Week 1**

The sage and thyme infuse the chicken in this dish with a light, beautiful aroma and flavor, and the vegetables add flavor, nutrients, and substance to round out the meal.

1 (4-pound) whole chicken

½ (¾-ounce) package fresh sage

½ (¾-ounce) package fresh thyme

1 medium sweet potato, cut into bite-size pieces

1 small yellow onion, sliced

1 cup halved Brussels sprouts

1 cup baby carrots

¼ cup coconut oil

Salt

Freshly ground black pepper

1. Preheat the oven to 375°F.
2. Place the chicken breast-side up in a 9-by-13-inch baking dish. Stuff most of the sage and thyme in the chicken cavity, leaving out 3 sprigs of each.
3. Scatter the sweet potato, onion, Brussels sprouts, carrots, and reserved sage and thyme sprigs around the chicken.
4. Add the unmelted coconut oil to the dish in 1-tablespoon dollops, and season with salt and pepper.
5. Transfer the dish to the oven, and bake until the thickest part of the chicken registers 180°F on a meat thermometer, 1½ to 2 hours. Remove from the oven.

Did you know? Instead of throwing out the chicken giblets when roasting a whole chicken, you can store them in a zip-top bag in the freezer to use the next time you're making Chicken Bone Broth (page 53). As you eat various pieces of the whole chicken, save those bones for the broth as well. They add flavor and nutrients to the broth, and that way, no part of the chicken is wasted.

Per Serving: Calories: 519; Total Fat: 36g; Saturated Fat: 18g; Sodium: 372mg; Carbohydrates: 13g; Fiber: 2g; Protein: 36g

Guilt-Free Turkey Burgers

GLUTEN-FREE, NUT-FREE, DAIRY-FREE, UNDER 30 MINUTES

SERVES 4 / PREP TIME: 5 MINUTES / COOK TIME: 15 MINUTES **Week 3**

When only a burger will do, these turkey burgers will fit the bill. Made with ground turkey and several herbs and spices, these burgers are tasty and healing to the gut. Cumin, which is a member of the parsley family, aids in digestion and can reduce IBS symptoms.

1 pound ground turkey

¼ bunch fresh cilantro, chopped

2 garlic cloves, minced

1 teaspoon ground cumin

½ teaspoon salt

¼ teaspoon freshly ground black pepper

2 tablespoons olive oil

1. In a large bowl, combine the turkey, cilantro, garlic, cumin, salt, and pepper, and mix well with your hands.
2. Shape the mixture into 4 even-size patties.
3. In a large skillet, heat the oil over medium heat.
4. Add the patties and cook until cooked through, about 7 minutes per side.

Substitution tip: Instead of ground turkey, you can use ground chicken.

Per Serving: Calories: 195; Total Fat: 8g; Saturated Fat: 1g; Sodium: 347mg; Carbohydrates: 1g; Fiber: 0g; Protein: 28g

Skillet Turkey Sausage and Sweet Potatoes

GLUTEN-FREE, NUT-FREE, DAIRY-FREE, ONE-POT

SERVES 4 / PREP TIME: 10 MINUTES / COOK TIME: 30 TO 40 MINUTES Week 4

You can have a breakfast ready in no time with this tasty recipe. Olive oil contains large amounts of antioxidants and has a pleasant, buttery flavor that mixes well with the other flavors in this dish. Thyme is thought to have antibacterial, insecticidal, and possibly antifungal properties.

⅓ cup olive oil, plus
2 tablespoons, divided

2 large sweet potatoes, chopped

¼ teaspoon salt

¼ teaspoon freshly ground
black pepper

1 small yellow onion, diced

1 pound bulk turkey sausage

2 tablespoons fresh thyme

1 teaspoon ground cumin

1. In a large skillet, heat ⅓ cup of oil over medium-high heat.
2. Add the sweet potatoes, salt, and pepper, and cook until the sweet potatoes are soft, 20 to 25 minutes. Transfer to a large bowl.
3. In the same pan, heat the remaining 2 tablespoons of oil over medium heat.
4. Add the onion, sausage, thyme, and cumin, and cook until the sausage has cooked through, 10 to 15 minutes.
5. Add the turkey mixture to the sweet potatoes and stir.

Substitution tip: For an even sweeter complement to the meal, swap out the yellow onion for ½ cup chopped shallots.

Per Serving: Calories: 506; Total Fat: 40g; Saturated Fat: 8g; Sodium: 638mg; Carbohydrates: 24g; Fiber: 4g; Protein: 16g

Baked Turkey with Honey and Thyme

GLUTEN-FREE, NUT-FREE, DAIRY-FREE, ONE-POT, 5 INGREDIENTS OR LESS

SERVES 4 / PREP TIME: 5 MINUTES / COOK TIME: 35 MINUTES **Week 2**

The combination of honey and thyme cooking in the oven will have your house smelling calm and delightful. This recipe is a great alternative to a large Thanksgiving turkey, but split turkey breasts can be found to enjoy year-round as well. Juicy, moist, slightly sweet with an herbal flair—you are bound to love this dish.

3 (1-pound) boneless, skinless turkey breasts

4 carrots, chopped

½ cup water

⅓ cup honey, or more if desired

2 teaspoons chopped fresh thyme

1. Preheat the oven to 400°F.
2. Put the turkey breasts in a 9-by-13-inch baking dish.
3. Put the carrots in a small bowl, and add the water, honey, and thyme. Stir with a fork to coat.
4. Pour the carrot mixture over the turkey breasts.
5. Transfer the dish to the oven, and roast until the turkey has cooked through, 30 to 35 minutes. Remove from the oven.

Did you know? Slow-cooking food is very healthy and optimal for gut healing because the food is contained in a sealed chamber to help keep moisture and nutrients in the food. To cook a boneless turkey breast in a slow cooker, simply place it in the slow cooker and add the water. Scatter the carrots around the turkey and spread the honey and thyme evenly over the turkey breast. Cover and cook on High for 1 hour, then turn to Low and cook until the thickest part of the breast registers 180°F on a meat thermometer, for about 3 hours.

Per Serving: Calories: 502; Total Fat: 2g; Saturated Fat: 0g; Sodium: 208mg; Carbohydrates: 30g; Fiber: 2g; Protein: 85g

Turkey and Sweet Potato Casserole

GLUTEN-FREE, DAIRY-FREE, ONE-POT

SERVES 6 / PREP TIME: 10 MINUTES / COOK TIME: 1 HOUR 5 MINUTES **Week 3**

Both a breakfast and dinner option, this casserole mixes sweet and savory. It includes marjoram, which has an earthy flavor profile and has been known to help with digestive issues from nausea to stomach cramps.

3 large sweet potatoes, chopped

**½ cup olive oil, plus
1 tablespoon, divided**

1 pound ground turkey

6 large eggs

½ cup full-fat coconut milk

1½ cups sliced mushrooms

**2 tablespoons chopped fresh
flat-leaf parsley**

**2 tablespoons chopped fresh
marjoram**

1 teaspoon salt

**½ teaspoon freshly ground
black pepper**

1. Preheat the oven to 350°F.
2. In a 9-by-13-inch baking dish, mix the sweet potatoes and ½ cup of olive oil.
3. Transfer the dish to the oven, and bake for 30 minutes.
4. Meanwhile, in a large skillet, heat the remaining 1 tablespoon of oil over medium heat.
5. Add the ground turkey, and cook until cooked through, 5 to 7 minutes.
6. While the sweet potatoes and turkey are cooking, in a medium bowl, whisk together the eggs and coconut milk, then stir in the mushrooms, parsley, marjoram, salt, and pepper.
7. Add the cooked turkey to the egg mixture.
8. Once the sweet potatoes have been in the oven for 30 minutes, remove the pan from the oven and pour the egg and turkey mixture into the baking dish. Return it to the oven, and bake until a toothpick inserted into the center comes out clean, for another 30 to 35 minutes. Remove from the oven.
9. Cut the casserole into squares and serve.

Substitution tip: If you are sensitive to mushrooms, simply omit them from this recipe. And if you enjoy an even stronger marjoram-flavored casserole, add an extra tablespoon.

Per Serving: Calories: 472; Total Fat: 37g; Saturated Fat: 11g; Sodium: 570mg; Carbohydrates: 16g; Fiber: 3g; Protein: 22g

LEMON AND DILL BROILED SALMON, PAGE 106

CHAPTER SEVEN

Seafood Mains

Lemon-Pepper Tuna

GLUTEN-FREE, NUT-FREE, DAIRY-FREE, UNDER 30 MINUTES, ONE-POT

SERVES 4 / PREP TIME: 5 MINUTES **Week 1**

Here's a quick way to add omega-3 proteins to your weekly meal plan. A can of lemon-pepper tuna contains far too many unnecessary ingredients and won't deliver half the flavor this recipe will. Using real lemon and pepper provides authentic flavor, and turmeric adds another anti-inflammatory component. Eat it as is, toss it over Cucumber and Blueberry Summer Salad with Blueberry Vinaigrette (page 86), or serve it on top of a slice of Autoimmune Paleo Bread (page 56).

3 (5-ounce) cans albacore tuna in water, drained

Juice of 1 lemon

¼ cup olive oil

½ teaspoon ground turmeric

½ teaspoon freshly ground black pepper

Salt

In a medium bowl, combine the tuna, lemon juice, oil, turmeric, and pepper. Season with salt. Mix well with a fork.

Make ahead: Mix up this tuna when you have the time, then store it in an airtight container in the refrigerator until you're ready to eat it.

Per Serving: Calories: 236; Total Fat: 14g; Saturated Fat: 2g; Sodium: 94mg; Carbohydrates: 1g; Fiber: 0g; Protein: 27g

Macadamia-Crusted Salmon with Cream Sauce

GLUTEN-FREE, DAIRY-FREE, UNDER 30 MINUTES

SERVES 4 / PREP TIME: 5 MINUTES / COOK TIME: 15 MINUTES **Week 3**

Just a few simple ingredients turn basic salmon into a beautiful entrée. Macadamia nuts are loaded with antioxidants and are known to benefit overall digestive health thanks to their fiber content. Their natural buttery flavor also complements salmon well. A twist of honey gives this dish a flavor you'll adore.

For the salmon

¾ cup macadamia nuts, ground

¼ cup unsweetened almond milk (or non-soy plant-based milk of choice)

1 teaspoon honey

4 (4-ounce) wild salmon fillets

Salt

For the sauce

½ cup macadamia nuts, ground

¼ cup unsweetened almond milk (or non-soy plant-based milk of choice)

½ teaspoon honey

To make the salmon

1. Preheat the oven 400°F.
2. In a medium bowl, whisk together the nuts, milk, and honey.
3. Pat the salmon dry, then dip each fillet in the macadamia mixture to coat both sides.
4. Place the salmon fillets in a 9-by-13-inch baking dish. Season with salt.
5. Transfer the dish to the oven, and bake until cooked through, for 11 to 13 minutes. Remove from the oven.

To make the sauce

1. While the salmon is in the oven, in a blender, combine the nuts, almond milk, and honey. Blend until smooth.
2. Remove the salmon from the oven, and drizzle with the sauce.

Did you know? Salmon is a nutrient-dense, gut-healing powerhouse, with inflammation-reducing omega-3 fatty acids and vitamin D.

Per Serving: Calories: 424; Total Fat: 32g; Saturated Fat: 6g; Sodium: 130mg; Carbohydrates: 7g; Fiber: 3g; Protein: 30g

Lemon and Dill Broiled Salmon

GLUTEN-FREE, NUT-FREE, DAIRY-FREE, UNDER 30 MINUTES, ONE-POT

SERVES 4 / PREP TIME: 5 MINUTES / COOK TIME: 10 MINUTES Week 1

Lemon and dill are natural flavor complements to salmon, and both are good sources of vitamin C. Dill has also been known to help with bacterial overgrowth, which is common in those with leaky gut syndrome. This fresh-flavored salmon dish can be enjoyed frequently.

4 (4-ounce) salmon fillets

Juice of 1 lemon

1 tablespoon olive oil

¼ (¾-ounce) package fresh dill

1½ teaspoons chopped fresh flat-leaf parsley, divided into fourths

Salt

Freshly ground black pepper

1. Preheat the oven to broil.
2. Place the salmon fillets on a rimmed baking sheet. Drizzle evenly with the lemon juice and oil, and rub it in with your hands to coat.
3. Sprinkle each fillet with the dill and parsley. Season with salt and pepper.
4. Transfer the baking sheet to the oven, and broil until the fillets have cooked through, for 6 to 7 minutes. Remove from the oven.

Substitution tip: If you like salmon, this is a simple recipe to make a couple times a week. For variety, you can change up the herbs. Try basil, tarragon, rosemary, or thyme instead of or in addition to the dill and parsley.

Per Serving: Calories: 313; Total Fat: 17g; Saturated Fat: 3g; Sodium: 126mg; Carbohydrates: 3g; Fiber: 1g; Protein: 32g

Summer Paleo Shrimp Succotash

GLUTEN-FREE, NUT-FREE, DAIRY-FREE, UNDER 30 MINUTES, ONE-POT

SERVES 4 / PREP TIME: 10 MINUTES / COOK TIME: 20 MINUTES Week 2

In this Paleo version of the classic succotash, asparagus and summer squash stand in for the usual lima beans and corn. Like the original, garlic is used in this recipe. Garlic has many proven healing benefits, including natural detoxifying properties. Though this is a summer recipe, the ingredients can be found, and the recipe enjoyed, year-round.

½ cup olive oil

6 asparagus spears, trimmed and chopped

4 small yellow squash, chopped

3 garlic cloves, minced

2 red bell peppers, chopped

1 medium yellow onion, chopped

1 tablespoon chopped fresh thyme

1 (12-ounce) bag cooked medium shrimp, peeled and deveined

Juice of 3 lemons

Salt

Freshly ground black pepper

1. In a large skillet, heat the oil over medium-high heat.
2. Add the asparagus, squash, garlic, peppers, onion, and thyme and sauté until tender, for about 12 minutes.
3. Add the shrimp and lemon juice, and cook until the shrimp is heated through, for about 5 minutes. Season with salt and pepper. Remove from the heat.

Make ahead: If you like, let the dish cool, then store in an airtight container in the refrigerator. When you're ready to reheat, simply place in a microwave for about 30 seconds, or heat in a saucepan over medium heat until warmed through.

Per Serving: Calories: 360; Total Fat: 27g; Saturated Fat: 4g; Sodium: 247mg; Carbohydrates: 14g; Fiber: 4g; Protein: 21g

Baked Tilapia with Creamy Cilantro Sauce

GLUTEN-FREE, DAIRY-FREE, UNDER 30 MINUTES

SERVES 4 / PREP TIME: 10 MINUTES / COOK TIME: 15 MINUTES **Week 2**

Tilapia is rich in vitamins and minerals like niacin, vitamin B12, phosphorus, selenium, and potassium. Because it's a light, white fish, a creamy sauce pairs nicely with it. Cilantro and lime go great with tilapia, and the extra creaminess of this sauce creates an even more savory dish.

For the tilapia

4 (6-ounce) tilapia fillets

Juice of 1 lemon

3 tablespoons olive oil

Salt

Freshly ground black pepper

For the sauce

1 bunch fresh cilantro

Juice of 1 small lime

1 cup full-fat coconut milk

2 tablespoons coconut aminos

1 tablespoon grated fresh ginger

½ teaspoon ground turmeric

Salt

Freshly ground black pepper

To make the tilapia

1. Preheat the oven to 425°F.
2. Place the tilapia fillets in a 9-by-13-inch baking dish. Drizzle evenly with the lemon juice and oil, and rub it in with your hands to coat. Season with salt and pepper.
3. Transfer the dish to the oven, and bake until the fillets flake easily with a fork, for 10 to 15 minutes. Remove from the oven.

To make the sauce

4. While the fish is in the oven, in a blender, combine the cilantro, lime juice, coconut milk, coconut aminos, ginger, and turmeric. Season with salt and pepper. Blend until smooth.
5. Pour the sauce on top of the fillets.

Substitution tip: If you can't find tilapia, you can swap it out for catfish, trout, snapper, or bass.

Per Serving: Calories: 386; Total Fat: 27g; Saturated Fat: 15g; Sodium: 119mg; Carbohydrates: 7g; Fiber: 2g; Protein: 33g

Mint-Lime Shrimp in Avocado Boats

GLUTEN-FREE, NUT-FREE, DAIRY-FREE, UNDER 30 MINUTES, ONE-POT

SERVES 4 / PREP TIME: 10 MINUTES / COOK TIME: 5 MINUTES Week 2

This flavorful shrimp dish features avocados, which go nicely with lime, mint, and maple syrup. The "boats" mean less cleanup, since you serve right in the avocado shell.

4 avocados

4 tablespoons olive oil, divided

Juice of 3 small limes

¼ bunch fresh mint, chopped

2 tablespoons maple syrup

Salt

1 (1-pound) bag cooked baby shrimp

1. Cut each avocado in half lengthwise, and remove the pit. Scoop the flesh into a large bowl, and reserve the shells.
2. Add 2 tablespoons of oil, the lime juice, the mint, the maple syrup, and a pinch of salt to the avocado. Mash until completely combined.
3. In a large skillet, heat the remaining 2 tablespoons of oil over medium-high heat.
4. Add the shrimp, and cook until warmed through, for 3 to 5 minutes.
5. Transfer the shrimp to the avocado mixture and stir to combine, then divide the mixture evenly among the 8 avocado shells.

Did you know? Mint is known to help an upset stomach and improve digestion.

Per Serving: Calories: 555; Total Fat: 42g; Saturated Fat: 6g; Sodium: 465mg; Carbohydrates: 25g; Fiber: 13g; Protein: 28g

Honey-Garlic Baked Cod

GLUTEN-FREE, DAIRY-FREE, UNDER 30 MINUTES, ONE-POT

SERVES 4 / PREP TIME: 5 MINUTES / COOK TIME: 15 MINUTES Week 3

If you love a classic teriyaki flavor but don't want to use bottled sauce, you'll love this recipe. It's sweet and salty—and done in less than 20 minutes, so it's likely to become a new household favorite. Serve with sautéed greens, if you like.

3 garlic cloves, minced

¼ cup honey

¼ cup coconut aminos

2 tablespoons olive oil

4 (4-ounce) cod fillets

Salt

1. Preheat the oven to 400°F.
2. In a small bowl, whisk together the garlic, honey, coconut aminos, and oil.
3. Place the cod fillets in a 9-by-13-inch baking dish, and pour the honey-garlic mixture evenly over them.
4. Transfer the dish to the oven, and bake until the fillets flake easily with a fork, for 12 to 15 minutes. Remove from the oven. Season with salt and serve.

Did you know? Honey is used in many healing protocols as it contains nutrients instead of just empty sugar calories. If a high-quality honey is used, it will be rich with antioxidants. Honey is also a monosaccharide, which means that most people can digest it with ease.

Per Serving: Calories: 233; Total Fat: 8g; Saturated Fat: 1g; Sodium: 127mg; Carbohydrates: 21g; Fiber: 0g; Protein: 20g

Salmon Patties

GLUTEN-FREE, DAIRY-FREE, ONE-POT, UNDER 30 MINUTES

SERVES 6 / PREP TIME: 10 MINUTES / COOK TIME: 20 MINUTES **Week 1**

Instead of bread crumbs, these salmon patties use coconut flour as a binder. They can be eaten as is, dipped in Dijon mustard, or wrapped in lettuce leaves as a burger substitute.

1 (14¾-ounce) can salmon, drained

3 large eggs, beaten

1 celery stalk, chopped

½ small yellow onion, chopped

¼ cup coconut flour

3 tablespoons Dijon mustard

1 teaspoon dried dill

¼ teaspoon salt

3 tablespoons olive oil

1. In a large bowl, combine the salmon, eggs, celery, onion, flour, mustard, dill, and salt. Using a fork, break up the salmon, and mix everything together.
2. Form the mixture into 8 to 10 salmon patties.
3. In a large skillet, heat the oil over medium-high heat.
4. Working in batches if necessary, add the patties and cook until they are golden brown on the bottom, for 6 to 9 minutes.
5. Carefully flip the patties, and cook until the other side is golden brown, for 6 to 9 minutes. (Do not flip the patties until they are golden brown on the bottom or they could fall apart.) Remove from the heat.

Substitution tip: For a slightly sweeter flavor, fry the patties in unrefined coconut oil instead of olive oil.

Per Serving: Calories: 261; Total Fat: 16g; Saturated Fat: 4g; Sodium: 321mg; Carbohydrates: 8g; Fiber: 5g; Protein: 21g

"Cheesy" Tuna Casserole

GLUTEN-FREE, DAIRY-FREE

SERVES 4 / PREP TIME: 10 MINUTES / COOK TIME: 1 HOUR 5 MINUTES Week 4

This dish is hearty like a traditional casserole but low in carbohydrates and high in omega-3 fatty acids, fiber, and vitamin B12 via the nutritional yeast. This is a complete meal the whole family will enjoy.

1 medium spaghetti squash, quartered and seeded

7 tablespoons olive oil, divided

2 large egg yolks

Juice of 1 lemon

¼ teaspoon salt

2 (5-ounce) cans albacore tuna in water, drained

¾ cup full-fat coconut milk

⅓ cup nutritional yeast, plus more for serving

1. Preheat the oven to 375°F.
2. Place the squash cut-side up in a 9-by-13-inch baking dish. Drizzle 1 tablespoon of oil on top.
3. Transfer the dish to the oven, and bake until the squash is tender, for 40 minutes. Remove from the oven and set aside to slightly cool.
4. Increase the oven temperature to 425°F. Lightly coat a medium casserole dish with 1 tablespoon of oil.
5. Scrape out the spaghetti-like strands of the squash, and put them a bowl.
6. Add the egg yolks, the lemon juice, the remaining 5 tablespoons of oil, and the salt, and mix together with a fork.
7. Add the tuna, and stir.
8. Add the coconut milk and nutritional yeast, and stir.
9. Transfer the mixture to the prepared casserole dish. Place in the oven, and bake until lightly browned, for about 22 minutes. Remove from the oven, and sprinkle more nutritional yeast on top, if desired.

Did you know? Nutritional yeast—sometimes called "nooch"—is a common cheese substitute for vegans and those who are dairy-free. It comes in both flake and powdered forms and is available at most grocery stores in packages or in the bulk section.

Per Serving: Calories: 564; Total Fat: 41g; Saturated Fat: 14g; Sodium: 229mg; Carbohydrates: 24g; Fiber: 7g; Protein: 32g

Lemon-Garlic Scallops with Sautéed Swiss Chard

GLUTEN-FREE, NUT-FREE, DAIRY-FREE, UNDER 30 MINUTES, ONE-POT

SERVES 3 / PREP TIME: 5 MINUTES / COOK TIME: 15 MINUTES **Week 1**

Scallops are sustainable and delicious, and they cook in less than 10 minutes. Scallops and Swiss chard are both good sources of magnesium and potassium, which are critical for gut healing.

**¼ cup olive oil, plus
2 tablespoons, divided**

2 garlic cloves, minced

1 pound large scallops

Juice of 1 lemon

1 bunch Swiss chard, chopped

Salt

Freshly ground black pepper

1. In a large skillet, heat ¼ cup of oil over medium heat.
2. Add the garlic, and cook until fragrant, for about 1 minute.
3. Pat the scallops dry, and add them to the pan in a single layer, along with the lemon juice. Cook until a golden brown crust forms, for about 2 minutes.
4. Flip the scallops, and cook just until the sides turn opaque, for 2 to 3 minutes. Transfer to a plate.
5. In the same pan, heat the remaining 2 tablespoons of oil.
6. Add the chard, and sauté until soft, for 3 to 5 minutes.
7. Divide the chard among 3 plates, and top with the scallops. Season with salt and pepper.

Substitution tip: If you're looking for a more buttery flavor, fry the scallops in ghee instead of olive oil.

Per Serving: Calories: 389; Total Fat: 29g; Saturated Fat: 4g; Sodium: 342mg; Carbohydrates: 6g; Fiber: 1g; Protein: 27g

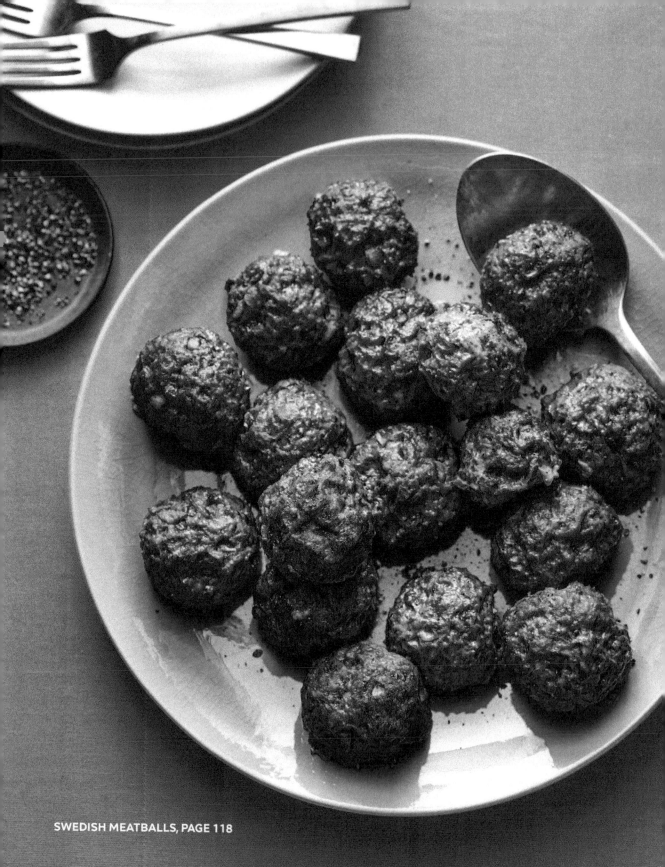

SWEDISH MEATBALLS, PAGE 118

CHAPTER EIGHT

Beef and Pork Mains

Honey-Ginger-Garlic Beef Stir-Fry

GLUTEN-FREE, DAIRY-FREE, UNDER 30 MINUTES, ONE-POT

SERVES 3 / PREP TIME: 5 MINUTES / COOK TIME: 25 MINUTES Week 2

Honey, ginger, and garlic form a triple healing powerhouse combination. Packed with natural antivirals and soothing properties, these three foods can do wonders for overall health and healing.

4 tablespoons coconut oil, divided

1¼ pounds lean beef stew meat

1 (12-ounce) bag broccoli florets

5 celery stalks, chopped

4 garlic cloves, minced

1 carrot, chopped

1 zucchini, chopped

¼ cup honey

2 tablespoons apple cider vinegar

4 teaspoons grated fresh ginger

Salt

Freshly ground black pepper

1. In a large skillet, heat 2 tablespoons of oil over medium-high heat.
2. Add the beef, and cook until browned on all sides and cooked through, about 10 minutes. Transfer to a plate.
3. In the same pan, heat the remaining 2 tablespoons of oil over medium-high heat.
4. Add the broccoli, celery, garlic, carrot, zucchini, honey, vinegar, and ginger. Season with salt and pepper. Cook, stirring frequently, until tender, for 10 minutes.
5. Return the beef to the pan, reduce the heat to medium, and cook until heated through and the flavors meld, for 5 minutes.

Substitution tip: If you don't want to have beef, you can use chicken or large shrimp instead.

Per Serving: Calories: 554; Total Fat: 26g; Saturated Fat: 19g; Sodium: 259mg; Carbohydrates: 76g; Fiber: 5g; Protein: 42g

Beef Burgers with Browned Shallots

GLUTEN-FREE, DAIRY-FREE, UNDER 30 MINUTES, ONE-POT

SERVES 4 / PREP TIME: 5 MINUTES / COOK TIME: 20 MINUTES Week 4

Fresh herbs and browned shallots make for a sweet and savory burger in this easy recipe. Just 3½ ounces of high-quality red meat gives the body more than 100 percent of the recommended daily intake for vitamin B12, which is essential for overall healing.

1 pound ground beef

1 garlic clove, minced

¼ large red onion, finely chopped

1 teaspoon chopped fresh rosemary

1 teaspoon chopped fresh thyme

¼ teaspoon salt

2 tablespoons coconut oil, divided

2 shallots, thinly sliced

1. In a large bowl, mix the beef, garlic, onion, rosemary, thyme, and salt with your hands.
2. Form the mixture into 4 equal-size patties.
3. In a large skillet, heat 1 tablespoon of oil over medium-high heat.
4. Add the patties, and cook until browned on both sides and cooked through, for 5 to 7 minutes per side. Transfer to a plate.
5. In the same pan, heat the remaining 1 tablespoon of oil over medium-high heat.
6. Add the shallots, and sauté until deep brown, for 3 to 5 minutes.
7. Top the burgers with the shallots.

Did you know? Shallots are in the same family as onions, leeks, scallions, and garlic. While they can be replaced with a regular onion, shallots have a more garlicky flavor.

Per Serving: Calories: 309; Total Fat: 24g; Saturated Fat: 13g; Sodium: 224mg; Carbohydrates: 2g; Fiber: 0g; Protein: 21g

Swedish Meatballs

GLUTEN-FREE, DAIRY-FREE, ONE-POT

SERVES 8 / PREP TIME: 10 MINUTES / COOK TIME: 35 MINUTES **Week 2**

Not only are meatballs delicious and filling, but this recipe includes ginger, which adds extra flavor and a gut-healing boost. These meatballs are great eaten on their own or tossed over spaghetti squash.

2 large eggs, beaten

¼ red onion, finely diced

1 teaspoon poultry seasoning

½ teaspoon grated fresh ginger

½ teaspoon ground allspice

½ teaspoon ground nutmeg

¼ teaspoon salt

¼ teaspoon freshly ground black pepper

2 pounds ground beef

1 cup unsweetened almond milk (or non-soy plant-based milk of choice)

1. Preheat the oven to 350°F. Line a rimmed baking sheet with parchment paper.
2. In a medium bowl, mix together the eggs, onion, poultry seasoning, ginger, allspice, nutmeg, salt, and pepper.
3. Add the ground beef and almond milk, and mix with your hands until well combined.
4. Form the mixture into about 16 meatballs, and place them on the prepared baking sheet.
5. Transfer the baking sheet to the oven, and bake until the meatballs have cooked through, for about 35 minutes (cut into one to check). Remove from the oven.

Make ahead: If desired, you can form the meatballs and freeze them on the baking sheet. Once they're frozen, pop them into a zip-top bag, and keep frozen until you are ready to bake them. Let them thaw for about 30 minutes, then bake.

Per Serving: Calories: 266; Total Fat: 19g; Saturated Fat: 8g; Sodium: 189mg; Carbohydrates: 1g; Fiber: 0g; Protein: 23g

Tomato and Basil No-Dough Pizza

GLUTEN-FREE, UNDER 30 MINUTES

SERVES 4 / PREP TIME: 15 MINUTES / COOK TIME: 15 MINUTES **Week 4**

Pizza night just took an interesting turn! This pizza's "crust" is formed with beef and coconut flour and flavored with oregano and garlic. The red sauce is a blend of sweet and spice, and the whole thing is topped with tomato, goat cheese, and olives for optimal gut healing.

For the sauce

1 (8-ounce) can no-salt-added tomato sauce

1 garlic clove, minced

2 tablespoons olive oil

1 tablespoon chopped fresh cilantro

1 tablespoon chopped fresh basil

1 teaspoon salt

⅛ teaspoon ground cumin

For the pizza

1 pound ground beef

3 tablespoons coconut flour

1 teaspoon dried oregano

½ teaspoon garlic powder

½ teaspoon salt

2 tablespoons olive oil

1 Roma tomato, sliced

1 (4-ounce) package goat cheese, sliced

1 (6-ounce) can sliced black olives, drained

2 tablespoons chopped fresh basil

To make the sauce

1. Preheat the oven to 350°F.
2. In a small saucepan, combine the tomato sauce, garlic, oil, cilantro, basil, salt, and cumin. Cook over low heat, stirring occasionally, until hot, for 5 to 7 minutes.

To make the pizza

1. Meanwhile, in a bowl, combine the beef, coconut flour, oregano, garlic powder, and salt. Mix well with your hands.
2. In a large oven-safe skillet, heat the oil over medium-high heat.
3. Carefully press the beef mixture into the bottom of the skillet to create a ½-inch-thick "crust." Cook until golden brown on the bottom, for about 3 minutes.
4. Using a large spatula, carefully flip the crust, and cook for 3 minutes. Remove from the heat.
5. Top the crust with the sauce, tomato, cheese, olives, and basil.
6. Transfer the pan to the oven, and bake until the cheese has melted and the toppings are warm, for 7 to 9 minutes. Remove from the oven.

Substitution tip: Instead of ground beef, you can use ground turkey or ground chicken for the "crust."

Per Serving: Calories: 609; Total Fat: 47g; Saturated Fat: 17g; Sodium: 1432mg; Carbohydrates: 17g; Fiber: 8g; Protein: 32g

"BLT"

GLUTEN-FREE, NUT-FREE, DAIRY-FREE, UNDER 30 MINUTES, ONE-POT

SERVES 4 / PREP TIME: 10 MINUTES / COOK TIME: 20 MINUTES Week 2

Beef, lettuce, and tomato—a brand-new way to BLT! This lettuce-wrapped burger also comes with an avocado boost. It's so full of flavor and healthy fats, you'll never miss a traditional bun or BLT again.

1 pound ground beef

¼ yellow onion, diced

1 teaspoon Dijon mustard

1 teaspoon garlic powder

½ teaspoon salt

¼ teaspoon freshly ground black pepper

2 tablespoons olive oil

8 butter lettuce leaves

1 tomato, thinly sliced

1 avocado, peeled, pitted, and thinly sliced

1. In a large bowl, combine the beef, onion, mustard, garlic powder, salt, and pepper. Mix well with your hands.
2. Form the mixture into 4 equal-size patties.
3. In a large skillet, heat the oil over medium-high heat.
4. Add the patties, and cook until cooked through, for 8 to 10 minutes per side.
5. Place each patty on a lettuce leaf, then add tomato slices and avocado slices, and top with another lettuce leaf.

Substitution tip: If you want to keep the B for bacon in this BLT, simply fry a few strips of regular or turkey bacon, and add them on top.

Per Serving: Calories: 383; Total Fat: 31g; Saturated Fat: 9g; Sodium: 385mg; Carbohydrates: 6g; Fiber: 4g; Protein: 22g

Mini Beef and Bacon Meatballs

GLUTEN-FREE, DAIRY-FREE

SERVES 4 / PREP TIME: 15 MINUTES / COOK TIME: 30 MINUTES **Week 4**

Almond meal, instead of bread crumbs, helps bind these mini meatballs perfectly. Serve these as part of a meal, or enjoy them as an appetizer.

2 tablespoons olive oil

4 bacon slices, trimmed of fat and chopped

1¼ pounds ground beef

1 celery stalk, diced

1 large egg, beaten

¾ cup almond meal

1 tablespoon chopped fresh sage

½ tablespoon chopped fresh thyme

½ teaspoon salt

½ teaspoon freshly ground black pepper

1. Preheat the oven to 350°F. Brush a 9-by-13-inch baking dish with the oil. Line a plate with a paper towel.
2. Heat a small skillet over low heat.
3. Add the bacon, and lightly fry for about 3 minutes. The bacon should be not quite done, since it will still be baked. Using a slotted spoon, transfer the bacon to drain on the paper towel.
4. In a large bowl, combine the beef, celery, egg, almond meal, sage, thyme, salt, and pepper.
5. Add the bacon, and mix with your hands.
6. Form the mixture into 16 meatballs. Place in the prepared baking dish.
7. Transfer the dish to the oven, and bake until the meatballs have cooked through, for about 30 minutes. Remove from the oven.

Per Serving: Calories: 588; Total Fat: 47g; Saturated Fat: 14g; Sodium: 532mg; Carbohydrates: 5g; Fiber: 3g; Protein: 38g

Pork Stir-Fry with Purple Cabbage

GLUTEN-FREE, DAIRY-FREE, UNDER 30 MINUTES, ONE-POT

SERVES 4 / PREP TIME: 5 MINUTES / COOK TIME: 25 MINUTES Week 3

This simple and delightful Asian-style recipe offers a large serving of purple cabbage, which is packed with vitamins C and K. Cabbage is known to keep inflammation in check and help improve digestion.

2 tablespoons coconut oil

1 small purple cabbage, thinly sliced

1 (8-ounce) package sliced mushrooms

1 pound ground pork

2 tablespoons coconut aminos

1 tablespoon apple cider vinegar

1 teaspoon garlic powder

1 teaspoon ground ginger

1 (10-ounce) bag baby spinach

Salt

Freshly ground black pepper

1. In a large skillet, heat the oil over medium-high heat.
2. Add the cabbage and cook until crisp-tender, for about 5 minutes.
3. Add the mushrooms and cook until slightly softened, for 2 minutes. Using tongs, transfer the cabbage and mushrooms to a plate.
4. Add the pork, coconut aminos, vinegar, garlic powder, and ginger to the same pan. Sauté until the pork is fully cooked, 7 to 10 minutes.
5. Add the baby spinach, and stir to wilt, for about 1 minute.
6. Return the cabbage and mushrooms to the pan, and cook until heated through, for 3 minutes. Season with salt and pepper.

Substitution tip: If you can't tolerate mushrooms, you can use shredded carrots instead.

Per Serving: Calories: 374; Total Fat: 24g; Saturated Fat: 12g; Sodium: 219mg; Carbohydrates: 17g; Fiber: 7g; Protein: 26g

One-Pan Turmeric Beef and Broccoli

GLUTEN-FREE, DAIRY-FREE, UNDER 30 MINUTES, ONE-POT

SERVES 4 / PREP TIME: 5 MINUTES / COOK TIME: 25 MINUTES **Week 3**

Beef and broccoli make up the majority of this dish, which is flavored with cilantro and the powerful spice turmeric. It's a beautiful yellow-tinted dish with a slight sweetness from the coconut aminos.

¼ cup olive oil, plus 1 tablespoon, divided

1 pound ground beef

1 (12-ounce) bag broccoli florets

6 scallions, chopped

¼ cup coconut aminos

1 tablespoon ground turmeric

½ cup chopped fresh cilantro

Salt

Freshly ground black pepper

1. In a large skillet, heat 1 tablespoon of oil over medium-high heat.
2. Add the beef, and sauté until cooked through, about 10 minutes. Using a slotted spoon, transfer to a plate.
3. In the same pan, heat the remaining ¼ cup of oil over medium-high heat.
4. Add the broccoli, scallions, coconut aminos, and turmeric, and sauté until the broccoli begins to brown, for 5 minutes.
5. Reduce the heat to medium, and sauté until the broccoli is tender, for 5 minutes.
6. Return the beef to the pan, add the cilantro, stir, and simmer until the flavors meld, for 3 minutes. Season with salt and pepper.

Substitution tip: Whenever a recipe in this book calls for coconut aminos, it can always be swapped out for tamari soy sauce if you prefer a saltier flavor.

Per Serving: Calories: 448; Total Fat: 35g; Saturated Fat: 10g; Sodium: 164mg; Carbohydrates: 12g; Fiber: 3g; Protein: 24g

Red-Wine Vinegar-Glazed Pork Chops with Peaches

GLUTEN-FREE, NUT-FREE, DAIRY-FREE, UNDER 30 MINUTES, ONE-POT

SERVES 4 / PREP TIME: 10 MINUTES / COOK TIME: 20 MINUTES Week 1

In this flavorful one-pot meal, the combination of red-wine vinegar, maple syrup, peaches, and thyme makes for a pork dish that's both savory and sweet. Red-wine vinegar and olive oil are both powerful antioxidants.

⅓ cup olive oil

⅓ cup red-wine vinegar

¼ cup maple syrup

4 (6-ounce) boneless pork chops

4 small peaches, pitted and quartered

½ (¾-ounce) package fresh thyme, chopped

Salt

Freshly ground black pepper

1. In a large skillet, heat the oil over medium-high heat.
2. Stir in the red-wine vinegar and maple syrup, then add the pork chops. Cook until the pork chops are browned on the bottom, 8 to 10 minutes.
3. Flip the pork chops over.
4. Add the peaches and thyme, and cook until the pork chops have cooked through, for 8 to 10 minutes. Season with salt and pepper.

Substitution tip: Not a fan of peaches, but still looking for a sweet fruit pairing? Try apples, nectarines, plums, or apricots.

Per Serving: Calories: 523; Total Fat: 33g; Saturated Fat: 8g; Sodium: 270mg; Carbohydrates: 29g; Fiber: 2g; Protein: 31g

Marinated Rosemary-Thyme Pork Loin

GLUTEN-FREE, NUT-FREE, DAIRY-FREE

SERVES 4 / PREP TIME: 5 MINUTES, PLUS 6 TO 8 HOURS TO MARINATE /

COOK TIME: 35 MINUTES Week 1

White balsamic vinegar becomes sweeter as it cooks, and it gives this pork loin a subtle sweetness. In addition to the vinegar, this pork loin is covered with the fragrant evergreen herb rosemary. Rosemary is often noted for improving digestion. Prepare this easy-to-make pork loin dish before heading to work or starting the day. Set it in the refrigerator, and when you're ready for dinner, place it in the oven. About 35 minutes later, dinner will be ready!

3 garlic cloves, minced

½ (¾-ounce) package fresh rosemary, chopped

5 tablespoons white balsamic vinegar

2 tablespoons olive oil

1 teaspoon dried thyme

1 (1-pound) pork loin, trimmed of silverskin

Salt

Freshly ground black pepper

1. In a small bowl, mix together the garlic, rosemary, vinegar, oil, and thyme.
2. Place the pork loin in a shallow baking dish, and prick it all over with a fork. Pour the marinade over it. Cover, and marinate in the refrigerator for 6 to 8 hours.
3. Preheat the oven to 450°F.
4. Place the dish in the oven, and bake the pork loin, turning halfway through, until it registers 145°F on a meat thermometer, for about 35 minutes. Season with salt and pepper.

Per Serving: Calories: 187; Total Fat: 10g; Saturated Fat: 2g; Sodium: 100mg; Carbohydrates: 1g; Fiber: 0g; Protein: 24g

SPAGHETTI SQUASH WITH BASIL AND
ARUGULA PESTO, PAGE 128

CHAPTER NINE

Vegetables and Sides

Spaghetti Squash with Basil and Arugula Pesto

GLUTEN-FREE, DAIRY-FREE, VEGAN

SERVES 2 / PREP TIME: 10 MINUTES / COOK TIME: 40 MINUTES **Week 3**

A traditional pesto is made with Parmesan cheese, but this recipe goes dairy-free and adds arugula and lemon to complement the basil. It also uses walnuts, which are high in omega-3 fatty acids, instead of pine nuts. The pesto is the perfect pairing for spaghetti squash, making for a creamy, delicious dish filled with healthy fats, vegetables, and herbs.

1 spaghetti squash, quartered and seeded

1 tablespoon olive oil, plus ½ cup, divided

1 cup raw walnuts

4 garlic cloves, chopped

Juice of 1 lemon

2 cups baby arugula

1½ cups fresh basil leaves

½ teaspoon salt

1. Preheat the oven to 375°F.
2. Place the squash cut-side up in a 9-by-13-inch baking dish. Drizzle 1 tablespoon of oil on top.
3. Transfer the dish to the oven, and bake until the squash is tender, for 35 to 40 minutes. Remove from the oven, and set aside to slightly cool.
4. Meanwhile, put the walnuts in a blender, and blend for 30 seconds.
5. Add the garlic, lemon juice, arugula, basil, salt, and ¼ cup of oil. Blend until almost completely blended.
6. Add the remaining ¼ cup of oil, and blend until smooth.
7. Scrape out the spaghetti-like strands of the squash, and put them a bowl. Pour the pesto on top.

Per Serving: Calories: 877; Total Fat: 86g; Saturated Fat: 11g; Sodium: 432mg; Carbohydrates: 31g; Fiber: 4g; Protein: 12g

Creamy Turmeric Veggies

GLUTEN-FREE, DAIRY-FREE, VEGAN, UNDER 30 MINUTES, ONE-POT

SERVES 4 / PREP TIME: 5 MINUTES / COOK TIME: 20 MINUTES Week 2

Creamy and gently spicy, these veggies can be served on their own or as an accompaniment to a main dish.

3 tablespoons coconut oil

1 (12-ounce) bag broccoli florets

2 summer squash, diced

1 tablespoon minced fresh ginger

1 garlic clove, minced

1 (13½-ounce) can full-fat coconut milk

4 teaspoons ground turmeric

Salt

Freshly ground black pepper

1. In a large skillet, heat the oil over medium-high heat.
2. Add the broccoli, squash, ginger, and garlic, and sauté until the vegetables soften, for 10 minutes.
3. Add the coconut milk and turmeric, cover, reduce the heat to medium, and simmer until creamy, for 10 minutes. Season with salt and pepper.

Substitution tip: Instead of coconut milk, you can use whatever plant-based milk you enjoy. This dish works well with almond milk and cashew milk.

Per Serving: Calories: 366; Total Fat: 34g; Saturated Fat: 29g; Sodium: 89mg; Carbohydrates: 17g; Fiber: 6g; Protein: 6g

Baked Kale Chips

GLUTEN-FREE, NUT-FREE, DAIRY-FREE, VEGAN, UNDER 30 MINUTES, ONE-POT, 5 INGREDIENTS OR LESS

SERVES 2 / PREP TIME: 5 MINUTES / COOK TIME: 20 MINUTES **Week 3**

The secret to crispy kale chips is that you must put the salt on them *after* they have baked. Baking them with the salt on can leave the kale limp and wilted. Kale is among the most nutrient-dense foods on the planet—one serving contains far more than 100 percent of the daily recommended value for vitamins A, K, and C. You'll want to eat these chips as often as possible!

1 bunch kale, tough stems removed and leaves torn into bite-size pieces

1 tablespoon olive oil

Salt

1. Preheat the oven to 350°F.
2. Put the kale leaves on a rimmed baking sheet, and drizzle with the oil. Use your hands to gently massage the kale leaves with the oil. Once they are fully coated, spread the leaves out in a single layer.
3. Transfer the baking sheet to the oven, and bake until the leaves are crisp, for 15 to 20 minutes. Remove from the oven. Season with salt.

Substitution tip: You can dress up kale chips however you want. After baking them, sprinkle with hemp seeds, sesame seeds, or whatever spices and herbs you like.

Per Serving: Calories: 159; Total Fat: 7g; Saturated Fat: 1g; Sodium: 165mg; Carbohydrates: 21g; Fiber: 2g; Protein: 6g

Roasted Brussels Sprouts and Walnuts

GLUTEN-FREE, DAIRY-FREE, VEGAN, UNDER 30 MINUTES, ONE-POT

SERVES 4 / PREP TIME: 5 MINUTES / COOK TIME: 20 MINUTES Week 4

This side dish pulls together the fresh fall flavors of Brussels sprouts, grapes, thyme, and walnuts, but it's a recipe that can be enjoyed year-round. Once the grapes have been baked, they soften and become even sweeter, providing a nice balance of sweet and salty.

4 cups Brussels sprouts, halved

2 cups red grapes

¼ cup raw walnuts, halved

2 tablespoons chopped fresh thyme

1 tablespoon olive oil

1½ teaspoons apple cider vinegar

½ teaspoon ground cinnamon

Salt

Freshly ground black pepper

1. Preheat the oven to 400°F.
2. In a medium bowl, toss together the Brussels sprouts, grapes, walnuts, thyme, oil, vinegar, and cinnamon. Season with salt and pepper. Spread out evenly on a large rimmed baking sheet.
3. Transfer the baking sheet to the oven, and bake until the grapes have softened and the Brussels sprouts are tender, for about 20 minutes.

Did you know? Many people drink a small amount of apple cider vinegar prior to eating protein-dense meals to help increase the acidity of the stomach.

Per Serving: Calories: 178; Total Fat: 9g; Saturated Fat: 1g; Sodium: 63mg; Carbohydrates: 24g; Fiber: 5g; Protein: 5g

Sweet and Spiced Sweet Potato Fries

GLUTEN-FREE, DAIRY-FREE, VEGAN, UNDER 30 MINUTES, ONE-POT

SERVES 4 / PREP TIME: 10 MINUTES / COOK TIME: 20 MINUTES Week 4

Preparing and making your own fries is simple, healthy, and healing. These are made with sweet potatoes instead of potatoes. Sweet potatoes are rich in vitamin A and contain a good amount of fiber per serving. Slightly sweet and mildly spiced, they are a perfect side dish for burger night.

2 large sweet potatoes

2½ tablespoons olive oil

1½ teaspoons coconut sugar

1½ teaspoon salt

1 teaspoon freshly ground black pepper

1 teaspoon paprika

½ teaspoon garlic powder

1. Preheat the oven to 425°F. Line a rimmed baking sheet with parchment paper.
2. Cut the sweet potatoes lengthwise into ½-inch-thick slabs, then cut each slab into ½-inch-thick fries.
3. Put the fries in a bowl, cover with water, and set aside for 3 minutes.
4. Drain the fries, and pat dry with a paper towel. Transfer to a zip-top bag. Add the oil, sugar, salt, pepper, paprika, and garlic powder. Seal, and shake vigorously until the fries are well coated.
5. Spread the fries in an even layer onto the prepared baking sheet.
6. Transfer the baking sheet to the oven, and bake for 10 minutes.
7. Flip the fries, return the baking sheet to the oven, and bake until slightly browned, for about 10 minutes. Remove from the oven.

Substitution tip: Feel free to replace the coconut sugar with stevia or monk fruit.

Per Serving: Calories: 150; Total Fat: 9g; Saturated Fat: 1g; Sodium: 809mg; Carbohydrates: 18g; Fiber: 2g; Protein: 1g

Creamy Mashed Cauliflower

GLUTEN-FREE, NUT-FREE, VEGETARIAN, UNDER 30 MINUTES, 5 INGREDIENTS OR LESS

SERVES 2 / PREP TIME: 10 MINUTES / COOK TIME: 20 MINUTES Week 3

Mashed cauliflower is a great swap for traditional mashed potatoes, to be served as a side dish for a protein or a base for a sauté. Baking the cauliflower in olive oil and then blending it with ghee yields a creamy texture.

1 head cauliflower, cut into small florets

2 tablespoons olive oil

¼ cup ghee

Salt

Freshly ground black pepper

1. Preheat the oven to 450°F.
2. Spread the cauliflower florets in a single layer onto a large rimmed baking sheet, and drizzle with the oil.
3. Transfer the baking sheet to the oven, and bake until the cauliflower easily breaks apart with a fork, for 18 to 20 minutes. Remove from the oven, and transfer to a blender.
4. Add the ghee, and blend until whipped together, about 3 minutes. Season with salt and pepper.

Did you know? Ghee (or clarified butter) is made by heating butter to remove the milk solids and water. It's great for those who typically cannot tolerate dairy, and it has been known to aid in digestion and help relieve inflammation. If you can't find ghee, try a cashew-based vegan butter or coconut yogurt in this recipe.

Per Serving: Calories: 378; Total Fat: 40g; Saturated Fat: 18g; Sodium: 118mg; Carbohydrates: 7g; Fiber: 3g; Protein: 3g

Sweet Potato and Butternut Squash Miso Mash

DAIRY-FREE, VEGAN, UNDER 30 MINUTES, ONE-POT

SERVES 4 / PREP TIME: 5 MINUTES / COOK TIME: 25 MINUTES **Week 2**

Here's a delicious substitute for mashed potatoes that includes miso for gut healing. Miso is a Japanese fermented soybean product that provides the gut with beneficial bacteria to help heal. Miso is salty; when combined with the sweetness of sweet potato, butternut squash, and coconut milk, its delicious flavor is a palate pleaser.

1 large sweet potato, peeled and diced

½ large butternut squash, peeled, seeded, and diced

2 teaspoons olive oil

Salt

¼ bunch fresh flat-leaf parsley, chopped

⅓ cup light coconut milk

2½ teaspoons miso paste

Freshly ground black pepper

1. Preheat the oven to 425°F.
2. Put the sweet potato and butternut squash in a 9-by-13-inch baking dish. Drizzle with the oil, and season with salt. Toss to coat, then spread out in a single layer.
3. Transfer the dish to the oven, and bake until you can easily pierce the sweet potato and squash with a fork, for about 25 minutes. Remove from the oven, and transfer to a large bowl.
4. Add the parsley, coconut milk, and miso. Season with pepper. Using an immersion blender, purée to a whipped consistency.

Did you know? Miso enhances many foods with the savory "umami" flavor, also known as "the fifth taste."

Per Serving: Calories: 131; Total Fat: 4g; Saturated Fat: 1g; Sodium: 203mg; Carbohydrates: 24g; Fiber: 4g; Protein: 3g

Kitchen Sink Vegetable Sauté

GLUTEN-FREE, DAIRY-FREE, VEGAN, UNDER 30 MINUTES, ONE-POT

SERVES 4 / PREP TIME: 10 MINUTES / COOK TIME: 20 MINUTES Week 4

This vegetable dish can include everything but the kitchen sink, so feel free to include any of your favorites. The vegetables chosen here are those that you could likely have left over from other meals during the 4-week meal plan.

⅓ cup olive oil

2 red bell peppers, chopped

1 small red onion, chopped

1 zucchini, chopped

1 yellow (summer) squash, chopped

1 medium sweet potato, chopped

1 garlic clove, minced

1 tablespoon chopped fresh thyme

1 tablespoon chopped fresh rosemary

⅓ cup coconut aminos

Salt

Freshly ground black pepper

1. In a large skillet, heat the oil over medium-high heat.
2. Add the bell peppers, onion, zucchini, squash, sweet potato, garlic, thyme, rosemary, and coconut aminos. Cook, stirring frequently, until tender, for 20 minutes. Season with salt and pepper.

Per Serving: Calories: 234; Total Fat: 17g; Saturated Fat: 3g; Sodium: 45mg; Carbohydrates: 20g; Fiber: 4g; Protein: 3g

Roasted Broccoli with Lemon Vinaigrette

GLUTEN-FREE, NUT-FREE, DAIRY-FREE, VEGAN, UNDER 30 MINUTES, ONE-POT, 5 INGREDIENTS OR LESS

SERVES 2 / PREP TIME: 5 MINUTES / COOK TIME: 20 MINUTES Week 2

Broccoli is not only filled with fiber but also acts as a prebiotic by feeding any beneficial bacteria the gut already has. Though broccoli can sometimes be hard to digest, cooking it with lemons aids digestion.

1 (12-ounce) bag broccoli florets

Juice of 2 lemons

2 tablespoons olive oil

Salt

Freshly ground black pepper

1. Preheat the oven to 450°F.
2. Put the broccoli florets on a rimmed baking sheet, and drizzle with the lemon juice and oil. Season with salt and pepper.
3. Transfer the baking sheet to the oven, and bake until golden brown around the edges, for about 20 minutes. Remove from the oven.

Did you know? The smaller your broccoli florets, the crispier they will turn out.

Per Serving: Calories: 184; Total Fat: 15g; Saturated Fat: 2g; Sodium: 138mg; Carbohydrates: 12g; Fiber: 5g; Protein: 5g

Maple-Balsamic Vinegar-Roasted Carrots

GLUTEN-FREE, NUT-FREE, DAIRY-FREE, VEGAN, UNDER 30 MINUTES

SERVES 3 / PREP TIME: 5 MINUTES / COOK TIME: 25 MINUTES **Week 1**

Carrots are one of the sweetest vegetables, and when you roast them with balsamic vinegar, maple syrup, and ground cinnamon, they get even sweeter. The ingredients in this dish are friendly for digestion and will satisfy your sweet tooth.

2 tablespoons olive oil

2 tablespoons white balsamic vinegar

2 tablespoons maple syrup

1 teaspoon ground cinnamon

1 pound carrots, cut into ¼-inch-thick slices

Salt

Freshly ground black pepper

1. Preheat the oven to 450°F.
2. In a large bowl, stir together the oil, vinegar, maple syrup, and cinnamon.
3. Add the carrots, and toss to mix well. Transfer to a rimmed baking sheet, and drizzle any leftover mixture over them. Spread out in a single layer, and season with salt and pepper.
4. Transfer the baking sheet to the oven, and bake until golden brown around the edges, for about 25 minutes. Remove from the oven.

Substitution tip: If you can find rainbow carrots, use them in this recipe for a bright, fun plate.

Per Serving: Calories: 181; Total Fat: 9g; Saturated Fat: 1g; Sodium: 156mg; Carbohydrates: 25g; Fiber: 4g; Protein: 1g

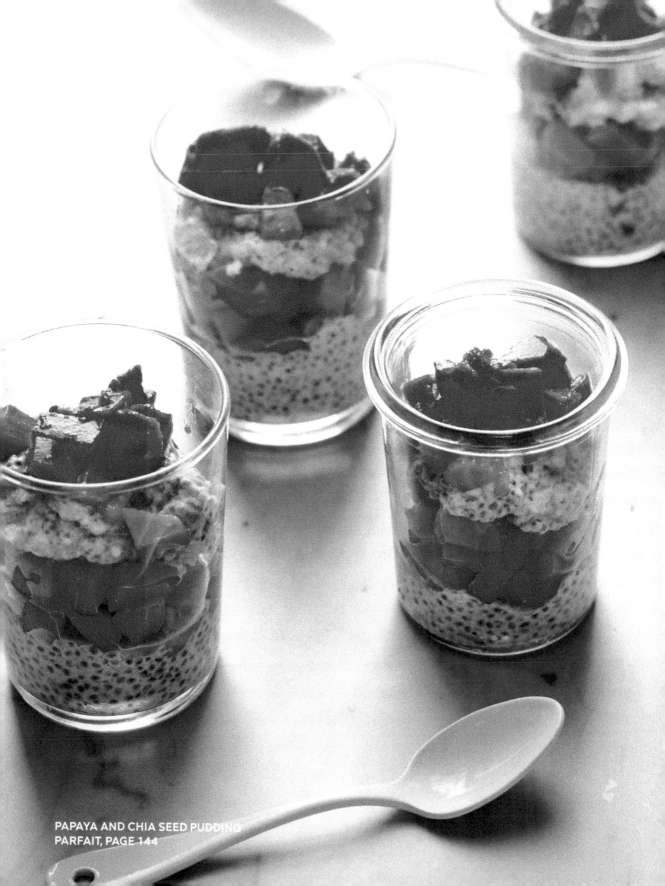

PAPAYA AND CHIA SEED PUDDING
PARFAIT, PAGE 144

CHAPTER TEN

Desserts

Banana-Coconut Cream Pudding

GLUTEN-FREE, DAIRY-FREE, ONE-POT

SERVES 2 / PREP TIME: 10 MINUTES, PLUS 4 HOURS TO SET Week 1

This thick, creamy pudding could become your favorite dessert. The gelatin is soothing for the gut lining.

2 medium bananas

1 egg yolk

1 cup full-fat coconut milk, divided

2 teaspoons vanilla extract

¼ teaspoon salt

1 tablespoon gelatin

1. In a medium bowl, combine the bananas, the egg yolk, ½ cup of coconut milk, the vanilla, and the salt. Blend with an immersion blender.
2. In a small pot, heat the remaining ½ cup of coconut milk over low heat until warm; don't allow it to bubble.
3. Add the heated milk to the banana mixture along with the gelatin. Stir until the gelatin has completely dissolved.
4. Put the bowl in the refrigerator until the pudding has set, for about 4 hours.

Did you know? According to the US Department of Agriculture, it's safe to ingest raw eggs as long as they are pasteurized. Most people who are intolerant of eggs have a problem with the white, not the yolk. If you can eat egg whites, use the leftover white from this recipe to make a quick omelet, tossing in another whole egg or two and chopped vegetables, as desired.

Per Serving: Calories: 432; Total Fat: 31g; Saturated Fat: 26g; Sodium: 321mg; Carbohydrates: 34g; Fiber: 6g; Protein: 8g

Nutty Chocolate Nice Cream

GLUTEN-FREE, DAIRY-FREE, VEGAN, UNDER 30 MINUTES, ONE-POT, 5 INGREDIENTS OR LESS

SERVES 2 / PREP TIME: 5 MINUTES, PLUS 15 MINUTES TO SET **Week 3**

Bananas, walnuts, chocolate, and a hint of vanilla create a flavorful "nice cream," which is an alternative to dairy ice cream. This dessert is an omega-3 fatty acid powerhouse, using both walnuts and walnut milk. The bananas and vanilla bring out the sweetness of the cocoa, which is a natural antioxidant.

2 large bananas, frozen

1 cup walnut milk

1 cup raw walnuts

¾ cup unsweetened cocoa powder

2 tablespoons vanilla extract

1. In a blender, combine the bananas, walnut milk, walnuts, cocoa powder, and vanilla. Blend until smooth.
2. Pour the mixture into a large bowl, and place in the freezer until set, about 15 minutes.

Substitution tip: Walnut milk is becoming very popular, but if you can't find it, use almond milk instead.

Per Serving: Calories: 656; Total Fat: 44g; Saturated Fat: 6g; Sodium: 189mg; Carbohydrates: 57g; Fiber: 21g; Protein: 18g

Mint-Lime Banana Shake

GLUTEN-FREE, DAIRY-FREE, VEGAN, UNDER 30 MINUTES, ONE-POT, 5 INGREDIENTS OR LESS

SERVES 2 / PREP TIME: 5 MINUTES **Week 4**

Tangy, creamy, and delicious, this shake puts a spin on any shake you've ever enjoyed. The apple and lime give it a little tang, while the banana and mint make it slightly sweet, creamy, and refreshing.

1 green apple, quartered

1 large banana, frozen

½ small lime, peeled

1 cup light coconut milk

½ cup ice cubes

1 tablespoon chopped fresh mint

In a blender, combine the apple, banana, lime, coconut milk, ice, and mint. Blend until smooth.

Substitution tip: If you love the taste of mint, add an extra tablespoon to this recipe for an even more refreshing flavor. Mint is great for digestion.

Per Serving: Calories: 203; Total Fat: 7g; Saturated Fat: 5g; Sodium: 42mg; Carbohydrates: 39g; Fiber: 5g; Protein: 1g

Chocolate-Cherry Cupcakes

GLUTEN-FREE, DAIRY-FREE, VEGETARIAN, UNDER 30 MINUTES, ONE-POT

SERVES 12 / PREP TIME: 10 MINUTES / COOK TIME: 20 MINUTES **Week 3**

Moist and delicious, these cupcakes offer a chunky treat. Chocolate and cherries are both natural antioxidants and can help reduce inflammation. You will love the classic chocolate-cherry combination in cupcake form!

½ cup almond flour

¼ cup unsweetened cocoa powder

5 tablespoons coconut sugar

1 teaspoon baking soda

½ teaspoon salt

2 large eggs

½ tablespoon almond extract

1 cup cherries, pitted

½ cup coconut oil, melted

1. Preheat the oven to 350°F. Line a standard muffin tin with cupcake liners.
2. In a small bowl, whisk together the almond flour, cocoa powder, coconut sugar, baking soda, and salt.
3. In a medium bowl, beat the eggs with the almond extract.
4. Add the cherries, and smash with a fork until the cherries are lumpy.
5. Add the dry mixture to the cherries, and stir to combine.
6. Add the melted coconut oil, and stir until a fudge-like batter forms.
7. Fill each cupcake liner about two-thirds of the way with the batter.
8. Transfer the muffin tin to the oven, and bake until a toothpick inserted into the center comes out clean, for 18 to 20 minutes. Remove from the oven.

Did you know? Almond meal (made from unblanched almonds) and almond flour (made from blanched almonds) are not the same thing. Almond meal is darker and has a gritty, grainy texture. Almond flour is lighter and has a softer flour-like texture.

Per Serving: Calories: 142; Total Fat: 12g; Saturated Fat: 8g; Sodium: 214mg; Carbohydrates: 9g; Fiber: 1g; Protein: 2g

Papaya and Chia Seed Pudding Parfait

GLUTEN-FREE, DAIRY-FREE, VEGAN, ONE-POT, 5 INGREDIENTS OR LESS

SERVES 1 / PREP TIME: 5 MINUTES, PLUS 4 HOURS TO SET Week 2

This tropical-inspired dessert is made with simple ingredients. The chia seeds contain fiber; they expand in the milk to form a pudding. Papaya is loaded with antioxidants and also contains an enzyme that makes protein easier to digest.

½ cup full-fat coconut milk

2½ tablespoons chia seeds

1 teaspoon stevia or monk fruit

1 papaya, peeled, seeded, and diced

1. In a small jar, combine the coconut milk, chia seeds, and stevia. Cover, and shake vigorously, then refrigerate until set, for about 4 hours.
2. In a parfait glass, layer the papaya and chia seed pudding.

Did you know? Even the seeds of the papaya are filled with nutrients, though they are bitter and would best be eaten separately from this dessert.

Per Serving: Calories: 516; Total Fat: 40g; Saturated Fat: 27g; Sodium: 37mg; Carbohydrates: 39g; Fiber: 17g; Protein: 9g

The Dirty Dozen and the Clean Fifteen™

A nonprofit environmental watchdog organization called Environmental Working Group (EWG) looks at data supplied by the US Department of Agriculture (USDA) and the Food and Drug Administration (FDA) about pesticide residues. Each year it compiles a list of the best and worst pesticide loads found in commercial crops. You can use these lists to decide which fruits and vegetables to buy organic to minimize your exposure to pesticides and which produce is considered safe enough to buy conventionally. This does not mean they are pesticide-free, though, so wash these fruits and vegetables thoroughly. The list is updated annually, and you can find it online at www.EWG.org/FoodNews.

Dirty Dozen™

1. Strawberries
2. Spinach
3. Kale
4. Nectarines
5. Apples
6. Grapes
7. Peaches
8. Cherries
9. Pears
10. Tomatoes
11. Celery
12. Potatoes

†Additionally, nearly three-quarters of hot pepper samples contained pesticide residues.

Clean Fifteen™

1. Avocados
2. Sweet corn
3. Pineapples
4. Sweet peas (frozen)
5. Onions
6. Papayas
7. Eggplants
8. Asparagus
9. Kiwis
10. Cabbages
11. Cauliflower
12. Cantaloupes
13. Broccoli
14. Mushrooms
15. Honeydew melons

Measurement Conversions

Volume Equivalents (Liquid)

US STANDARD	US STANDARD (OUNCES)	METRIC (APPROXIMATE)
2 tablespoons	1 fl. oz.	30 mL
¼ cup	2 fl. oz.	60 mL
½ cup	4 fl. oz.	120 mL
1 cup	8 fl. oz.	240 mL
1½ cups	12 fl. oz.	355 mL
2 cups or 1 pint	16 fl. oz.	475 mL
4 cups or 1 quart	32 fl. oz.	1 L
1 gallon	128 fl. oz.	4 L

Oven Temperatures

FAHRENHEIT	CELSIUS (APPROXIMATE)
250°F	120°C
300°F	150°C
325°F	165°C
350°F	180°C
375°F	190°C
400°F	200°C
425°F	220°C
450°F	230°C

Volume Equivalents (Dry)

US STANDARD	METRIC (APPROXIMATE)
⅛ teaspoon	0.5 mL
¼ teaspoon	1 mL
½ teaspoon	2 mL
¾ teaspoon	4 mL
1 teaspoon	5 mL
1 tablespoon	15 mL
¼ cup	59 mL
⅓ cup	79 mL
½ cup	118 mL
⅔ cup	156 mL
¾ cup	177 mL
1 cup	235 mL
2 cups or 1 pint	475 mL
3 cups	700 mL
4 cups or 1 quart	1 L

Weight Equivalents

US STANDARD	METRIC (APPROXIMATE)
½ ounce	15 g
1 ounce	30 g
2 ounces	60 g
4 ounces	115 g
8 ounces	225 g
12 ounces	340 g
16 ounces or 1 pound	455 g

References

Allbritton, Jen. "Eat Your Eggs and Have Your Chickens Too." The Weston A. Price Foundation. Last modified. April 3, 2009. https://www.westonaprice.org/health-topics/childrens-health/eat-your-eggs-and-have-your-chickens-too/.

DiMagno, E. P. "Regulation of Interdigestive Gastrointestinal Motility and Secretion." *Digestion* 58 (1997): 53–55. https://doi.org/10.1159/000201527.

Ehrlein, H. J., and M. Schemann. "Gastrointestinal Motility." Accessed October 6, 2019. http://humanbiology.wzw.tum.de/fileadmin/Bilder/tutorials/tutorial.pdf.

Irritable Bowel Syndrome Self Help and Support Group. "Migrating Motor Complex: SIBO & the Importance of Fasting." Accessed October 6, 2019. http://www.ibsgroup.org/forums/topic/179961-migrating-motor-complex-sibo-the-importance-of-fasting/.

Palsdottir, Hrefna. "Is Eating Raw Eggs Safe and Healthy?" *Healthline.* Last modified July 23, 2016. https://www.healthline.com/nutrition/eating-raw-eggs/.

Takahashi, Toku. "Mechanism of Interdigestive Migrating Motor Complex." *Journal of Neurogastroenterology and Motility* 18, 3 (July 2012): 246–57. https://doi.org/10.5056/jnm.2012.18.3.246

Index

About the Author

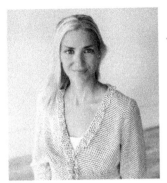

Sarah Kay Hoffman is a gut researcher and journalist who seeks out highly detailed information and then condenses it in digestible ways for women worldwide.

Sarah graduated from the University of Minnesota with a degree in marketing, English, and mass communications. After years of struggling with her own health issues and believing that there must be more to healing than the answers she was given, she went on to study at the Institute for Integrative Nutrition to become a certified health coach. She began devoting every minute to studying, researching, and practicing everything she could about gut health and gut healing.

Sarah founded the online community A Gutsy Girl (AGutsyGirl.com) in 2012 in order to connect with other women worldwide who were also seemingly sitting in silence about topics like IBS, IBD, and infertility and looking for reasonable approaches for healing.

When Sarah is not giving back to the Gutsy community, she can be found writing on a more personal level at *A Thyme for Milk and Honey* on Medium.com, creating beautiful things in the natural foods industry as marketing director at DELIGHTED BY Desserts, working out, traveling, drinking lattes, reading her Bible, and soaking up all the love that is her husband, three (very small) adorable children, family, and friends.

Printed in the USA
CPSIA information can be obtained
at www.ICGtesting.com
CBHW041032060524
8112CB00003B/13